Keto Air Fryer Cookbook for Beginners

Discover Delicious Low-Carb Recipes and Master the Art of Air Frying for Quick and Healthy Ketogenic Meals

By Xyla Winona

TABLE OF CONTENTS

Are you ready to explore the incredible versatility of your air fryer? Look no further! " Keto Air Fryer Cookbook for Beginners" is a comprehensive collection of delectable dishes that will take your air frying game to the next level. Whether you're a seasoned air fryer enthusiast or just starting, this cookbook is packed with various recipes to suit every taste and occasion.

In this cookbook, you'll find a wide range of appetizers, main courses, sides, snacks, and even desserts – all specially crafted for your air fryer. We've carefully selected 100 mouthwatering recipes that showcase the magic of air frying, giving you a healthier alternative to traditional deep frying without sacrificing taste or texture.

Discover the joy of crispy chicken tenders, zesty wings, and succulent shrimp skewers that are perfectly cooked and full of flavour. Indulge in cheesy appetizers, flavorful vegetable medleys, and innovative twists on classic favourites. From savoury meats to vegetarian delights, there's something for everyone in this collection.

But it doesn't stop there! "Keto Air Fryer Cookbook for Beginners" also offers tips and tricks to help you master your air fryer's settings, cooking times, and temperature adjustments. You'll learn how to achieve that irresistible golden crispness while keeping your dishes tender and juicy on the inside. Say goodbye to greasy, unhealthy meals and embrace the ease and health benefits of air frying.

Whether you're hosting a dinner party, preparing a quick weeknight meal, or simply looking for healthier snack options, this cookbook has you covered. With clear instructions, helpful tips, and stunning food photography, you'll be inspired to create culinary masterpieces that will impress your family and friends.

So, get ready to embark on an exciting culinary adventure with "Keto Air Fryer Cookbook for Beginners." It's time to elevate your cooking skills, enjoy delicious meals, and savour the benefits of healthier, air-fried dishes. Let the magic of your air fryer transform your kitchen and your taste buds.

CRISPY PARMESAN CHICKEN TENDERS

Prep Time: 15 minutes Cooking Time: 15 minutes Serving: 4

Ingredients:

- 1 pound chicken tenders
- 1 cup grated Parmesan cheese
- 1 cup almond flour
- Two teaspoons paprika
- One teaspoon of garlic powder
- One teaspoon of dried oregano
- One teaspoon of dried basil
- 1/2 teaspoon salt
- 1/4 teaspoon black pepper
- Two eggs, beaten
- Cooking spray

Directions:

1. Preheat your air fryer to 400°F (200°C).

2. In a shallow bowl, combine grated Parmesan cheese, almond flour, paprika, garlic powder, dried oregano, dried basil, salt, and black pepper. Mix well.

3. Dip each chicken tender into the beaten eggs, allowing any excess to drip off, then coat it thoroughly in the Parmesan mixture. Press the mixture onto the chicken to ensure a good coating.

4. Place the coated chicken tenders on a plate or tray.

5. Lightly spray the air fryer basket with cooking spray to prevent sticking.

6. Arrange the chicken tenders in a single layer in the air fryer basket, ensuring they are not touching.

7. Cook the chicken tenders in the air fryer for 8-10 minutes, flipping halfway through the cooking time. The chicken should be golden brown and crispy.

8. Remove the chicken tenders from the air fryer and let them cool for a few minutes before serving.

9. Serve the Crispy Parmesan Chicken Tenders with your favourite dipping sauce or as part of a meal. They make a great appetizer or main dish.

Nutrition Facts (per serving):

- Calories: 320
- Fat: 15g
- Protein: 37g
- Carbohydrates: 8g
- Fibre: 3g
- Sugar: 1g
- Sodium: 640mg

Note: Nutrition facts may vary depending on the specific ingredients and brands used.

ZESTY LEMON PEPPER WINGS

Prep Time: 10 minutes Cooking Time: 40 minutes Serving: 4 servings

Ingredients:

- 2 pounds of chicken wings
- Two tablespoons of olive oil
- Two teaspoons of lemon zest
- One tablespoon of freshly squeezed lemon juice
- One teaspoon of black pepper
- One teaspoon salt

- One teaspoon of garlic powder
- One teaspoon of onion powder
- 1/2 teaspoon paprika
- 1/2 teaspoon dried oregano
- 1/4 teaspoon cayenne pepper (optional, for some heat)
- Fresh parsley, chopped (for garnish)

Directions:

1. Preheat your oven to 400°F (200°C). Line a baking sheet with parchment paper or aluminium foil for easy cleanup.

2. In a large bowl, combine the olive oil, lemon zest, lemon juice, black pepper, salt, garlic powder, onion powder, paprika, dried oregano, and cayenne pepper (if using). Mix well to create a marinade.

3. Add the chicken wings to the bowl and toss them in the marinade until evenly coated. Allow the wings to marinate for about 10 minutes, or refrigerate them for up to 1 hour for more flavour.

4. Arrange the chicken wings on the prepared baking sheet in a single layer, ensuring they're not touching each other too closely.

5. Place the baking sheet in the preheated oven and bake the wings for 20 minutes. Then, flip the wings over and bake for an additional 15-20 minutes or until they're cooked through and crispy.

6. Once the wings are done, remove them from the oven and let them cool for a few minutes. Sprinkle them with freshly chopped parsley for added freshness and colour.

7. Serve the zesty lemon pepper wings hot as an appetizer or as part of a main course. They pair well with a dipping sauce like ranch dressing or blue cheese dressing. Enjoy!

Nutrition Facts (per serving):

- Calories: 350
- Fat: 25g
- Saturated Fat: 6g
- Cholesterol: 95mg
- Sodium: 650mg
- Carbohydrates: 2g
- Fibre: 0g
- Sugar: 0g
- Protein: 28g

Note: Nutrition facts are approximate and may vary depending on the ingredients used.

GARLIC BUTTER SHRIMP SKEWERS

Prep Time: 15 minutes Cooking Time: 10 minutes Serving: 4

Ingredients:

- 1 pound (450g) large shrimp, peeled and deveined
- Four cloves garlic, minced
- 1/4 cup (56g) unsalted butter, melted
- Two tablespoons fresh parsley chopped
- One tablespoon of lemon juice
- Salt and pepper to taste
- Wooden skewers, soaked in water for 30 minutes

Directions:

1. Preheat your grill or stovetop grill pan to medium-high heat.
2. In a small bowl, combine the minced garlic, melted butter, chopped parsley, lemon juice, salt, and pepper. Mix well to combine.

3. Thread the shrimp onto the soaked wooden skewers, piercing each shrimp through the tail and the thickest part of the body.

4. Brush the garlic butter mixture generously over the shrimp skewers, coating them evenly on both sides.

5. Place the shrimp skewers on the preheated grill or grill pan and cook for about 2-3 minutes per side or until the shrimp turn pink and opaque. Be careful not to overcook them, as they can become rubbery.

6. Once cooked, remove the shrimp skewers from the grill and transfer them to a serving plate.

7. Serve the Garlic Butter Shrimp Skewers hot, garnished with additional chopped parsley, if desired.

Nutrition Facts (per serving):

- Calories: 230
- Total Fat: 14g
- Saturated Fat: 8g
- Cholesterol: 270mg
- Sodium: 280mg
- Total Carbohydrate: 2g

- Dietary Fiber: 0g
- Sugars: 0g
- Protein: 23g

Enjoy your delicious Garlic Butter Shrimp Skewers!

SPICY BUFFALO CAULIFLOWER BITES

Prep Time: 15 minutes Cooking Time: 25 minutes Serving: 4 servings

Ingredients:

- One large cauliflower head cut into florets
- 1/2 cup all-purpose flour
- 1/2 cup water
- One teaspoon of garlic powder
- 1/2 teaspoon paprika
- 1/2 teaspoon salt
- 1/4 teaspoon black pepper
- 1/4 cup hot sauce
- Two tablespoons unsalted butter melted
- One tablespoon honey (optional, for a touch of sweetness)

- Ranch or blue cheese dressing for serving
- Celery sticks for serving

Directions:

1. Preheat your oven to 450°F (230°C). Line a baking sheet with parchment paper or lightly grease it.

2. In a large bowl, whisk together the flour, water, garlic powder, paprika, salt, and black pepper to make a batter. The consistency should be smooth and slightly thick.

3. Dip each cauliflower floret into the batter, coating it evenly, and then place it on the prepared baking sheet. Repeat this process until all the florets are coated.

4. Bake the cauliflower in the preheated oven for 20-25 minutes or until golden brown and crispy. Flip the florets halfway through the baking time to ensure even cooking.

5. While the cauliflower is baking, prepare the buffalo sauce. In a small bowl, mix the hot sauce, melted butter, and honey (if using). Adjust the amount of hot sauce according to your desired level of spiciness.

6. Once the cauliflower is cooked, remove it from the oven and let it cool for a few minutes. Then, transfer the baked florets to a large mixing bowl.

7. Pour the buffalo sauce over the cauliflower and toss gently until the florets are evenly coated.

8. Serve the Spicy Buffalo Cauliflower Bites with ranch or blue cheese dressing on the side, along with celery sticks.

Nutrition Facts (per serving):

- Calories: 150
- Fat: 5g
- Saturated Fat: 3g
- Cholesterol: 10mg
- Sodium: 800mg
- Carbohydrates: 25g
- Fibre: 4g
- Sugar: 6g
- Protein: 4g

Enjoy your Spicy Buffalo Cauliflower Bites! They make delicious appetizers or snacks.

BACON-WRAPPED JALAPENO POPPERS

Prep Time: 20 minutes Cooking Time: 20 minutes Serving: 10 poppers

Ingredients:

- Five jalapeno peppers
- Five slices of bacon, cut in half
- 4 ounces cream cheese, softened
- 1/2 cup shredded cheddar cheese
- 1/2 teaspoon garlic powder
- 1/4 teaspoon paprika
- Salt and pepper to taste

Directions:

1. Preheat your oven to 400°F (200°C) and line a baking sheet with parchment paper.
2. Cut the jalapeno peppers in half lengthwise and remove the seeds and membranes. You can use a spoon to scrape them out.
3. In a mixing bowl, combine the softened cream cheese, shredded cheddar cheese, garlic powder, paprika, salt, and pepper. Mix until well combined.

4. Spoon the cream cheese mixture into the jalapeno pepper halves, filling them evenly.

5. Wrap each stuffed jalapeno half with a bacon slice half. Secure the bacon with toothpicks if needed.

6. Place the bacon-wrapped jalapeno poppers on the prepared baking sheet.

7. Bake in the preheated oven for about 20 minutes or until the bacon is crispy and the peppers are tender.

8. Once cooked, remove the jalapeno poppers from the oven and let them cool for a few minutes.

9. Serve the bacon-wrapped jalapeno poppers warm as an appetizer or snack.

Nutrition Facts (per serving): Calories: 136 Total Fat: 12g

- Saturated Fat: 6g
- Trans Fat: 0g Cholesterol: 32mg Sodium: 247mg Total Carbohydrate: 2g
- Dietary Fiber: 0g
- Sugars: 1g Protein: 6g

Enjoy your delicious Bacon-Wrapped Jalapeno Poppers!

HERB-ROASTED PORK TENDERLOIN

Prep Time: 15 minutes Cooking Time: 25 minutes Serving: 4 servings

Ingredients:

- 1 ½ pounds pork tenderloin
- Two tablespoons of olive oil
- Two cloves garlic, minced
- One tablespoon of chopped fresh rosemary
- One tablespoon of chopped fresh thyme
- One teaspoon of dried oregano
- One teaspoon salt
- ½ teaspoon black pepper

Directions:

1. Preheat the oven to 425°F (220°C).
2. In a small bowl, combine the minced garlic, chopped rosemary, chopped thyme, dried oregano, salt, and black pepper.
3. Pat the pork tenderloin dry with paper towels. Rub the olive oil all over the pork tenderloin.

4. Sprinkle the herb mixture evenly over the pork tenderloin, pressing it onto the surface to adhere.

5. Heat a large oven-safe skillet over medium-high heat. Once the skillet is hot, add the pork tenderloin and sear it on all sides until browned, about 2 minutes per side.

6. Transfer the skillet with the pork tenderloin to the preheated oven. Roast for about 20-25 minutes or until the internal temperature reaches 145°F (63°C) for medium-rare or 160°F (71°C) for medium.

7. Remove the pork tenderloin from the oven and let it rest for about 5 minutes before slicing.

8. Slice the herb-roasted pork tenderloin into ½-inch thick slices. Serve warm, and enjoy!

Nutrition Facts (per serving):

- Calories: 275
- Total Fat: 11g
- Saturated Fat: 2.5g
- Cholesterol: 105mg
- Sodium: 600mg

- Carbohydrates: 1g
- Fibre: 0g
- Sugars: 0g
- Protein: 39g

Note: Nutrition facts are approximate and may vary depending on the ingredients used.

MEDITERRANEAN EGGPLANT FRIES

Prep Time: 15 minutes Cooking Time: 20 minutes Serving: 4 servings

Ingredients:

- Two medium eggplants
- 1/2 cup all-purpose flour
- One teaspoon of garlic powder
- One teaspoon of dried oregano
- 1/2 teaspoon salt
- 1/4 teaspoon black pepper
- Two large eggs, beaten
- 1 cup breadcrumbs
- Olive oil for frying
- Lemon wedges for serving

Directions:

1. Preheat the oven to 400°F (200°C).

2. Slice the eggplants into long, thin strips resembling fries.

3. Mix the flour, garlic powder, dried oregano, salt, and black pepper in a shallow dish.

4. Dip each eggplant strip into the flour mixture, coating it evenly, then dip it into the beaten eggs, and finally coat it with breadcrumbs. Repeat this process until all the eggplant strips are coated.

5. Heat a large skillet over medium heat and add enough olive oil to cover the bottom.

6. Working in batches, fry the coated eggplant strips until golden brown and crispy, about 2-3 minutes per side. Place the fried eggplant on a paper towel-lined plate to drain excess oil.

7. Transfer the fried eggplant to a baking sheet and bake in the preheated oven for an additional 10 minutes to ensure they are fully cooked and crispy.

8. Remove from the oven and serve the Mediterranean eggplant fries hot with lemon wedges on the side.

Nutrition Facts (per serving):

- Calories: 220
- Fat: 8g
- Saturated Fat: 1g
- Cholesterol: 93mg
- Sodium: 427mg
- Carbohydrates: 31g
- Fibre: 7g
- Sugar: 7g
- Protein: 8g

Note: The nutrition facts are approximate and may vary based on the specific ingredients used.

CRUNCHY COCONUT SHRIMP

Prep Time: 15 minutes Cooking Time: 15 minutes Serving: 4 servings

Ingredients:

- 1 pound large shrimp, peeled and deveined
- 1 cup all-purpose flour
- One teaspoon salt
- 1/2 teaspoon black pepper

- 1/2 teaspoon paprika
- 1/4 teaspoon cayenne pepper (optional for added heat)
- Two large eggs
- 1 cup shredded coconut
- Vegetable oil for frying
- Sweet chilli sauce for dipping

Directions:

1. In a shallow bowl, combine the all-purpose flour, salt, black pepper, paprika, and cayenne pepper. Set aside.
2. In another bowl, beat the eggs.
3. Place the shredded coconut in a separate bowl.
4. Dip each shrimp into the flour mixture, shaking off any excess.
5. Next, dip the shrimp into the beaten eggs, allowing any excess to drip off.
6. Roll the shrimp in the shredded coconut, pressing gently to adhere the coconut to the shrimp.
7. Heat vegetable oil in a large skillet or deep fryer to about 350°F (175°C).

8. Fry the coated shrimp in batches for 2-3 minutes per side or until they turn golden brown and crispy.

9. Remove the shrimp from the oil using a slotted spoon and place them on a paper towel-lined plate to drain excess oil.

10. Serve the Crunchy Coconut Shrimp hot with sweet chilli sauce for dipping.

Nutrition Facts (per serving):

- Calories: 280
- Total Fat: 12g
- Saturated Fat: 8g
- Cholesterol: 220mg
- Sodium: 650mg
- Total Carbohydrate: 26g
- Dietary Fiber: 2g
- Sugars: 2g
- Protein: 17g

Enjoy your Crunchy Coconut Shrimp!

BBQ PULLED PORK SLIDERS

Prep Time: 15 minutes Cooking Time: 8 hours Serving: 6 sliders

Ingredients:

- 2 pounds (900g) of boneless pork shoulder
- One tablespoon of brown sugar
- One teaspoon paprika
- One teaspoon of garlic powder
- One teaspoon of onion powder
- One teaspoon salt
- 1/2 teaspoon black pepper
- 1 cup barbecue sauce
- 1/4 cup apple cider vinegar
- 1/4 cup chicken broth
- Six slider buns
- Coleslaw (optional for serving)

Directions:

1. Mix the brown sugar, paprika, garlic powder, onion powder, salt, and black pepper in a small bowl to make a dry rub.

2. Rub the dry rub all over the pork shoulder, ensuring it is evenly coated. Place the pork shoulder in a slow cooker.

3. In a separate bowl, combine the barbecue sauce, apple cider vinegar, and chicken

broth. Pour the sauce mixture over the pork shoulder in the slow cooker.

4. Cover the slow cooker and cook on low heat for 8 hours or until the pork is tender and easily shreds with a fork.

5. Once the pork is cooked, remove it from the slow cooker and transfer it to a cutting board. Use two forks to shred the pork.

6. Return the shredded pork to the slow cooker and stir it into the sauce until well coated. Let it cook for 15-30 minutes on low heat to absorb the flavours.

7. Toast the slider buns if desired. Place a generous amount of the pulled pork on each bun.

8. Serve the BBQ-pulled pork sliders with coleslaw on top, if desired. Enjoy!

Nutrition Facts (per serving):

- Calories: 380
- Fat: 12g
- Saturated Fat: 4g
- Cholesterol: 95mg
- Sodium: 970mg
- Carbohydrates: 38g

- Fibre: 2g
- Sugar: 17g
- Protein: 30g

Note: The nutrition facts may vary depending on the specific brands of ingredients used and any additional toppings or modifications.

CHEESY BROCCOLI TOTS

Prep Time: 15 minutes Cooking Time: 25 minutes Serving: 4 servings

Ingredients:
- 2 cups broccoli florets
- 1 cup shredded cheddar cheese
- 1/4 cup grated Parmesan cheese
- 1/4 cup breadcrumbs
- Two cloves garlic, minced
- 1/4 teaspoon salt
- 1/4 teaspoon black pepper
- Two eggs, lightly beaten

Directions:

1. Preheat your oven to 400°F (200°C) and line a baking sheet with parchment paper.

2. Steam the broccoli florets until tender, about 5 minutes. Drain well and chop into small pieces.

3. In a large bowl, combine the chopped broccoli, shredded cheddar cheese, grated Parmesan cheese, breadcrumbs, minced garlic, salt, and black pepper. Mix well to combine.

4. Add the beaten eggs to the broccoli mixture and stir until all ingredients are evenly distributed.

5. Take a tablespoonful of the mixture and shape it into a tot shape using your hands. Place it on the prepared baking sheet. Repeat with the remaining mixture.

6. Bake the tots in the preheated oven for 20-25 minutes or until golden brown and crispy.

7. Remove from the oven and let them cool for a few minutes before serving.

Nutrition Facts (per serving):

- Calories: 180

- Fat: 11g
- Carbohydrates: 10g
- Protein: 12g
- Fibre: 2g
- Sugar: 2g
- Sodium: 400mg

Enjoy your Cheesy Broccoli Tots!

Garlic Parmesan Brussels Sprouts

Prep Time: 10 minutes Cooking Time: 25 minutes Serving: 4 servings

Ingredients:

- 1 pound Brussels sprouts
- two tablespoons of olive oil
- three cloves garlic, minced
- 1/4 cup grated Parmesan cheese
- Salt and pepper to taste

Directions:

1. Preheat your oven to 400°F (200°C). Line a baking sheet with parchment paper or aluminium foil.

2. Trim the ends of the Brussels sprouts and remove any yellowed or damaged outer leaves. Cut each Brussels sprout in half.

3. In a large bowl, combine the Brussels sprouts, olive oil, minced garlic, Parmesan cheese, salt, and pepper. Toss until the Brussels sprouts are evenly coated.

4. Transfer the Brussels sprouts to the prepared baking sheet and spread them out in a single layer.

5. Roast the Brussels sprouts in the preheated oven for about 20-25 minutes or until they are tender and lightly browned. Stir or shake the baking sheet halfway through cooking to ensure even browning.

6. Remove the Brussels sprouts from the oven and transfer them to a serving dish. Sprinkle with additional grated Parmesan cheese, if desired.

7. Serve the Garlic Parmesan Brussels Sprouts as a side dish or a tasty appetizer. Enjoy!

Nutrition Facts (per serving):

• Calories: 120
• Fat: 7g
• Carbohydrates: 10g
• Fiber: 4g
• Protein: 6g

Note: Nutrition facts may vary depending on the specific ingredients and brands used.

ITALIAN MEATBALLS

Prep Time: 20 minutes Cooking Time: 30 minutes Servings: 4

Ingredients:

• 1 pound ground beef
• 1/2 pound ground pork
• 1/2 cup bread crumbs
• 1/4 cup grated Parmesan cheese
• 1/4 cup chopped fresh parsley
• 1/4 cup milk
• 1 small onion, finely chopped

- 2 cloves garlic, minced
- 1 teaspoon dried oregano
- one teaspoon of dried basil
- 1/2 teaspoon salt
- 1/4 teaspoon black pepper
- 1 large egg
- 2 cups marinara sauce

Directions:

1. Preheat the oven to 375°F (190°C). Line a baking sheet with parchment paper.

2. In a large bowl, combine the ground beef, ground pork, bread crumbs, Parmesan cheese, parsley, milk, onion, garlic, oregano, basil, salt, pepper, and egg. Mix well until all the ingredients are evenly incorporated.

3. Shape the meat mixture into golf ball-sized meatballs and place them on the prepared baking sheet.

4. Bake the meatballs in the preheated oven for 20-25 minutes or until they are cooked through and browned on the outside.

5. While the meatballs are baking, heat the marinara sauce in a large skillet over medium heat.

6. Once the meatballs are cooked, transfer them to the skillet with the marinara sauce. Gently stir to coat the meatballs in the sauce.

7. Reduce the heat to low and let the meatballs simmer in the sauce for 5 minutes, allowing the flavours to meld together.

8. Serve the Italian meatballs hot with your choice of pasta or crusty bread. They can also be served as a sandwich filling or as an appetizer with toothpicks.

Nutrition Facts (per serving):

• Calories: 350
• Total Fat: 22g
• Saturated Fat: 8g
• Cholesterol: 115mg
• Sodium: 650mg
• Total Carbohydrate: 13g
• Dietary Fiber: 2g
• Sugars: 5g
• Protein: 25g

Enjoy your delicious Italian meatballs

CRISPY AVOCADO FRIES

Prep Time: 15 minutes Cooking Time: 15 minutes Serving: 2-4 servings

Ingredients:

• two large avocados
• 1 cup all-purpose flour
• two large eggs, beaten
• 1 cup breadcrumbs

- 1/2 teaspoon salt
- 1/2 teaspoon paprika
- 1/4 teaspoon black pepper
- Cooking oil for frying

Directions:

1. Preheat the oven to 200°C (400°F). Line a baking sheet with parchment paper and set aside.

2. Cut the avocados in half lengthwise, remove the pit, and peel off the skin. Slice each avocado half into thick wedges.

3. place the flour, beaten eggs, and breadcrumbs in three separate shallow bowls.

4. Season the breadcrumbs with salt, paprika, and black pepper. Mix well to combine.

5. Dip each avocado wedge into the flour, coating it completely. Shake off any excess flour.

6. Next, dip the floured avocado wedge into the beaten eggs, allowing any excess to drip off.

7. Finally, coat the avocado wedge with the seasoned breadcrumbs, pressing gently to ensure they stick. Repeat the process with all the avocado wedges.

8. Heat cooking oil in a deep skillet or pot over medium-high heat. The oil should be hot but not smoking.

9. Carefully place a few avocado wedges into the hot oil, making sure not to overcrowd the

pan. Fry for 2-3 minutes on each side or until golden brown and crispy. Remove the fried avocado wedges from the oil and place them on a paper towel-lined plate to drain excess oil. 10. Once all the avocado wedges are fried, transfer them to the prepared baking sheet and place them in the oven for an additional 5 minutes to ensure they are heated through.

11. Serve the crispy avocado fries immediately with your favourite dipping sauce, such as spicy mayo, salsa, or ranch dressing.

Nutrition Facts (per serving):

• Calories: 250
• Total Fat: 14g
• Saturated Fat: 2g
• Cholesterol: 93mg
• Sodium: 425mg
• Carbohydrates: 26g
• Fiber: 7g
• Sugar: 2g
• Protein: 7g

Enjoy your crispy avocado fries!

TERIYAKI SALMON FILLETS

Prep Time: 10 minutes Cooking Time: 15 minutes Serving: 4

Ingredients:

- four salmon fillets
- 1/4 cup soy sauce
- two tablespoons of honey
- 2 tablespoons rice vinegar
- 1 tablespoon sesame oil
- two cloves garlic, minced
- one teaspoon of grated ginger
- one tablespoon of cornstarch
- two tablespoons of water
- Sesame seeds (for garnish)
- Sliced green onions (for garnish)
- Steamed rice (optional)

Directions:

1. Preheat the oven to 400°F (200°C). Line a baking sheet with parchment paper or foil and set aside.

2. In a small bowl, whisk together the soy sauce, honey, rice vinegar, sesame oil, minced garlic, and grated ginger.

3. Place the salmon fillets in a shallow dish or a zip-top bag. Pour the teriyaki marinade over the salmon, coating each fillet evenly. Allow the salmon to marinate for about 10 minutes.

4. While the salmon is marinating, prepare the teriyaki sauce. In a small saucepan, combine the cornstarch and water, stirring until the cornstarch is dissolved. Add the remaining marinade from the dish or bag to the saucepan and heat over medium heat. Cook the sauce,

stirring constantly, until it thickens. Remove from heat and set aside.

5. Transfer the marinated salmon fillets onto the prepared baking sheet, skin-side down. Discard the remaining marinade.

6. Bake the salmon in the preheated oven for about 12-15 minutes or until the fish is cooked and flakes easily with a fork.

7. Remove the salmon from the oven and brush each fillet with the prepared teriyaki sauce. Return the salmon to the oven and broil for 2-3 minutes or until the sauce caramelizes slightly.

8. Remove the salmon from the oven and let it rest for a few minutes. Sprinkle with sesame seeds and sliced green onions for garnish.

9. Serve the teriyaki salmon fillets hot, with steamed rice if desired. Enjoy!

Nutrition Facts (per serving):
• Calories: 300
• Fat: 15g
• Protein: 30g
• Carbohydrates: 12g
• Fiber: 1g
• Sugar: 9g
• Sodium: 750mg

Please note that the nutrition facts may vary depending on the specific ingredients and brands used.

CAJUN SEASONED SWEET POTATO WEDGES

Prep Time: 10 minutes Cooking Time: 25 minutes Serving: 4

Ingredients:

- two large sweet potatoes
- 2 tablespoons olive oil
- one teaspoon of paprika
- one teaspoon of garlic powder
- one teaspoon of onion powder
- 1/2 teaspoon cayenne pepper
- 1/2 teaspoon dried thyme
- 1/2 teaspoon dried oregano
- 1/2 teaspoon salt
- 1/4 teaspoon black pepper

Directions:

1. Preheat the oven to 425°F (220°C). Line a baking sheet with parchment paper or lightly grease it.

2. Wash the sweet potatoes thoroughly and cut them into wedges, leaving the skin on.

3. In a large bowl, combine olive oil, paprika, garlic powder, onion powder, cayenne pepper, dried thyme, dried oregano, salt, and black pepper. Stir well to make a Cajun seasoning blend.

4. Add the sweet potato wedges to the bowl and toss them with the Cajun seasoning mixture until evenly coated.

5. Arrange the seasoned sweet potato wedges in a single layer on the prepared baking sheet.

6. Place the baking sheet in the preheated oven and bake for about 25 minutes or until the sweet potatoes are tender and golden brown, flipping them once halfway through the cooking time.

7. Remove from the oven and let the Cajun-seasoned sweet potato wedges cool for a few minutes before serving.

Nutrition Facts (per serving):
- Calories: 180
- Total Fat: 7g
- Saturated Fat: 1g
- Sodium: 325mg
- Total Carbohydrate: 27g
- Dietary Fiber: 4g
- Sugars: 6g
- Protein: 2g

Note: The nutrition facts are approximate and may vary based on the specific ingredients used.

STUFFED PORTOBELLO MUSHROOMS

Prep Time: 15 minutes Cooking Time: 25 minutes Servings: 4

Ingredients:

- four large Portobello mushrooms
- one tablespoon of olive oil
- 1 small onion, finely chopped
- two cloves garlic, minced
- 1 cup fresh spinach, chopped
- 1 cup breadcrumbs
- 1/2 cup grated Parmesan cheese
- 1/4 cup chopped fresh parsley
- Salt and pepper to taste

Directions:

1. Preheat your oven to 375°F (190°C).
2. Remove the stems from the Portobello mushrooms and gently scrape out the gills using a spoon. Set the mushroom caps aside.
3. heat the olive oil over medium heat in a large skillet. Add the chopped onion, minced garlic, and sauté until the onion becomes translucent and fragrant.
4. Add the chopped spinach to the skillet and cook until wilted. Remove from heat.
5. In a bowl, combine the breadcrumbs, grated Parmesan cheese, chopped parsley, salt, and pepper. Mix well.
6. Add the cooked spinach mixture to the breadcrumb mixture and stir until everything is well combined.

7. Spoon the stuffing mixture into the Portobello mushroom caps, filling them evenly.

8. Place the stuffed mushrooms on a baking sheet lined with parchment paper.

9. Bake in the preheated oven for about 25 minutes or until the mushrooms are tender and the stuffing is golden brown.

10. Once cooked, remove from the oven and let them cool slightly before serving.

11. Serve the stuffed Portobello mushrooms as a main course or a delicious appetizer.

Nutrition Facts (per serving):

- Calories: 180
- Total Fat: 8g
- Saturated Fat: 3g
- Cholesterol: 8mg
- Sodium: 380mg
- Total Carbohydrate: 20g
- Dietary Fiber: 3g
- Sugars: 4g
- Protein: 9g

Note: The nutrition facts are approximate and may vary based on the specific ingredients and quantities used.

BACON-WRAPPED ASPARAGUS BUNDLES

Prep Time: 15 minutes Cooking Time: 20 minutes Servings: 4

Ingredients:

- 1 pound (450g) asparagus spears, tough ends trimmed
- eight slices of bacon
- two tablespoons of olive oil
- Salt and pepper to taste

Directions:

1. Preheat your oven to 400°F (200°C) and line a baking sheet with parchment paper.
2. Divide the asparagus spears into eight equal bundles.
3. Take a slice of bacon and wrap it tightly around one bundle of asparagus, starting at the bottom and spiralling it up to the top. Repeat with the remaining asparagus bundles and bacon slices.
4. Place the bacon-wrapped asparagus bundles on the prepared baking sheet, seam side down.
5. Drizzle the olive oil over the bundles, then season with salt and pepper to taste.
6. Bake in the preheated oven for 15-20 minutes or until the bacon is crispy and the asparagus is tender. You can also broil for the last 1-2 minutes to get the bacon extra crispy.
7. Remove from the oven and let the bundles cool for a few minutes before serving.

Nutrition Facts (per serving):

- Calories: 180
- Fat: 13g
- Carbohydrates: 4g
- Fiber: 2g
- Protein: 11g

Enjoy your delicious Bacon-Wrapped Asparagus Bundles!

LEMON HERB ROASTED CHICKEN THIGHS

Prep Time: 15 minutes Cooking Time: 40 minutes Servings: 4

Ingredients:

- eight chicken thighs, bone-in and skin-on
- two lemons, juiced and zested
- three tablespoons of olive oil
- four cloves garlic, minced
- one tablespoon of fresh thyme leaves
- one tablespoon of fresh rosemary leaves, chopped
- one teaspoon of salt
- 1/2 teaspoon black pepper

Directions:

1. Preheat the oven to 425°F (220°C). Line a baking sheet with parchment paper or foil for easy cleanup.
2. In a small bowl, whisk together the lemon juice, lemon zest, olive oil, minced garlic,

thyme leaves, rosemary, salt, and black pepper.

3. Place the chicken thighs on the prepared baking sheet. Pour the lemon herb marinade over the chicken thighs, and coat them evenly on all sides.

4. Massage the marinade into the chicken thighs, ensuring they are well coated. Let them marinate for at least 10 minutes to allow the flavours to develop.

5. Roast the chicken thighs in the preheated oven for about 40 minutes or until the internal temperature reaches 165°F (74°C). If desired, you can broil the chicken for 2-3 minutes at the end to achieve a crispy skin.

6. Once cooked, remove the chicken thighs from the oven and let them rest for a few minutes before serving.

7. Serve the lemon herb roasted chicken thighs with your choice of side dishes, such as roasted vegetables, rice, or a fresh salad.

Nutrition Facts (per serving):
- Calories: 350
- Fat: 25g
- Protein: 28g
- Carbohydrates: 4g
- Fiber: 1g
- Sugar: 1g
- Sodium: 600mg

Note: The nutrition facts provided are approximate and may vary based on the specific ingredients and serving size used.

MOZZARELLA STICKS WITH MARINARA SAUCE

Prep Time: 15 minutes Cooking Time: 15 minutes Servings: 4
Ingredients:
- eight mozzarella cheese sticks
- 1 cup all-purpose flour
- two large eggs, beaten
- 2 cups breadcrumbs
- one teaspoon of dried Italian seasoning
- 1/2 teaspoon garlic powder
- 1/2 teaspoon salt
- Vegetable oil for frying

For the Marinara Sauce:
- one can (14 ounces) of crushed tomatoes
- 2 cloves garlic, minced
- one teaspoon of dried basil
- one teaspoon of dried oregano
- 1/2 teaspoon sugar
- Salt and pepper to taste

Directions:
1. Preheat the vegetable oil in a deep fryer or a large pot to 375°F (190°C).

2. In three separate shallow bowls, set up a breading station. In the first bowl, place the all-purpose flour. In the second bowl, beat the eggs. In the third bowl, combine the breadcrumbs, dried Italian seasoning, garlic powder, and salt.

3. Cover one mozzarella stick in the flour, shaking off any excess. Dip it into the beaten eggs, ensuring it is fully coated. Then, roll it in the breadcrumb mixture, pressing gently to adhere the breadcrumbs to the cheese. Place the coated mozzarella stick on a baking sheet and repeat the process with the remaining cheese sticks.

4. Once all the mozzarella sticks are coated, place them in the preheated oil and fry them for about 2-3 minutes or until they turn golden brown. Be sure not to overcrowd the fryer or pot; fry them in batches if needed.

5. While the mozzarella sticks are frying, prepare the marinara sauce. In a small saucepan, combine the crushed tomatoes, minced garlic, dried basil, dried oregano, sugar, salt, and pepper. Cook the sauce over medium heat, stirring occasionally, for about 5 minutes or until heated through.

6. Once the mozzarella sticks are golden brown, remove them from the oil using a

slotted spoon or tongs. Place them on a paper towel-lined plate to drain any excess oil.

7. Serve the hot mozzarella sticks with the marinara sauce on the side for dipping. Enjoy!

Nutrition Facts (per serving): Calories: 285 Total Fat: 13g Saturated Fat: 7g Cholesterol: 98mg Sodium: 711mg Total Carbohydrate: 24g Dietary Fiber: 2g Sugar: 3g Protein: 17g

Note: The nutrition facts provided are approximate values and may vary based on the specific ingredients used.

GREEK CHICKEN SOUVLAKI SKEWERS

Prep Time: 15 minutes Cooking Time: 10 minutes Serving: 4 servings

Ingredients:

• 1.5 lbs (680 g) boneless, skinless chicken breast cut into bite-sized pieces
• 1/4 cup olive oil
• 1/4 cup lemon juice
• two tablespoons Greek yoghurt
• three cloves garlic, minced
• one tablespoon dried oregano
• one teaspoon dried thyme
• one teaspoon dried rosemary
• one teaspoon salt
• 1/2 teaspoon black pepper

- one red bell pepper, cut into chunks
- one green bell pepper, cut into chunks
- one red onion, cut into chunks
- four pita breads
- Tzatziki sauce for serving (optional)

Directions:

1. In a bowl, whisk together the olive oil, lemon juice, Greek yoghurt, minced garlic, dried oregano, dried thyme, rosemary, salt, and black pepper.

2. Add the chicken pieces to the marinade and toss until they are well-coated. Allow the chicken to marinate for at least 30 minutes or up to 4 hours in the refrigerator.

3. Preheat your grill or grill pan over medium-high heat.

4. Thread the marinated chicken pieces onto skewers, alternating with the bell peppers and red onion chunks.

5. Place the skewers on the preheated grill and cook for about 4-5 minutes per side or until the chicken is cooked through and has nice grill marks.

6. While the chicken is cooking, warm the pita bread on the grill for about 1 minute per side.

7. Remove the skewers from the grill and allow them to rest for a few minutes.

8. Serve the Greek chicken souvlaki skewers with warm pita loaves of bread and tzatziki sauce, if desired.

Nutrition Facts (per serving): Calories: 340 Total Fat: 12g

• Saturated Fat: 2g

• Trans Fat: 0g Cholesterol: 95mg Sodium: 660mg Total Carbohydrate: 24g

• Dietary Fiber: 3g

• Sugars: 4g Protein: 34g

Note: Nutrition facts may vary depending on the specific brands and quantities of ingredients used.

PARMESAN ZUCCHINI CHIPS

Prep Time: 15 minutes Cooking Time: 25 minutes Serving: 4 servings

Ingredients:

• two large zucchini

• 1/2 cup grated Parmesan cheese

• 1/2 cup breadcrumbs

• one teaspoon garlic powder

• 1/2 teaspoon paprika

• 1/2 teaspoon salt

• 1/4 teaspoon black pepper

• two large eggs, beaten

• Cooking spray

Directions:

1. Preheat your oven to 425°F (220°C). Line a baking sheet with parchment paper and set aside.

2. Cut the zucchini into thin slices, about 1/4-inch thick. Pat the slices dry with a paper towel to remove any excess moisture.

3. In a shallow bowl, combine the grated Parmesan cheese, breadcrumbs, garlic powder, paprika, salt, and black pepper. Mix well.

4. Dip each zucchini slice into the beaten eggs, making sure to coat both sides.

5. Then, press each slice into the Parmesan breadcrumb mixture, ensuring that both sides are evenly coated. Place the coated zucchini slices on the prepared baking sheet in a single layer.

6. Lightly spray the zucchini slices with cooking spray. This will help them become crispy in the oven.

7. Bake in the preheated oven for about 20-25 minutes or until the zucchini chips are golden brown and crispy. Flip the chips halfway through the cooking time to ensure even browning.

8. Once the chips are done, remove them from the oven and let them cool slightly before serving.

Nutrition Facts (per serving):

- Calories: 138
- Fat: 6g
- Carbohydrates: 13g
- Fiber: 2g
- Protein: 9g
- Sodium: 652mg

Note: The nutrition facts are approximate and may vary based on the specific ingredients and quantities used.

RANCH SEASONED POTATO WEDGES

Prep Time: 10 minutes Cooking Time: 30 minutes Serving: 4 servings

Ingredients:
- four large potatoes
- two tablespoons olive oil
- one tablespoon ranch seasoning mix
- Salt, to taste
- Freshly ground black pepper, to taste
- Chopped fresh parsley for garnish (optional)

Directions:

1. Preheat your oven to 425°F (220°C). Line a baking sheet with parchment paper or lightly grease it.

2. Wash the potatoes thoroughly and pat them dry with a clean kitchen towel.

3. Cut each potato into wedges. Start by cutting the potato in half lengthwise, then cut each half into thirds or fourths; depending on the size of the potato bowl, combine the olive oil and ranch seasoning in a large bowl mix. Toss the potato wedges in the mix, ensuring they are evenly coated.

5. Arrange the seasoned potato wedges in a single layer on the prepared baking sheet. Sprinkle with salt and freshly ground black pepper to taste.

6. Place the baking sheet in the preheated oven and bake for about 25-30 minutes, or until the wedges are golden brown and crispy, flipping them halfway through the cooking time.

7. Once cooked, remove the potato wedges from the oven and let them cool for a few minutes. Garnish with chopped fresh parsley, if desired.

8. Serve the Ranch Seasoned Potato Wedges hot as a side dish or appetizer. They go well with ketchup, ranch dressing, or your favourite dipping sauce.

Nutrition Facts (per serving):
- Calories: 215
- Fat: 7g
- Carbohydrates: 36g
- Fiber: 4g
- Protein: 4g

- Sodium: **360mg**

Note: Nutritional values are approximate and may vary depending on the ingredients used.

Enjoy your Ranch Seasoned Potato Wedges!

PESTO STUFFED CHICKEN BREAST

Prep Time: 15 minutes Cooking Time: 25 minutes Servings: 4

Ingredients:
- four boneless, skinless chicken breasts
- 1/2 cup basil pesto
- four slices mozzarella cheese
- Salt and pepper, to taste
- one tablespoon olive oil

Directions:
1. Preheat your oven to 400°F (200°C).
2. Using a sharp knife, make a horizontal slit in each chicken breast to create a pocket for the stuffing. Be careful not to cut all the way through.
3. Season the chicken breasts with salt and pepper, both inside and out.
4. Spoon approximately two tablespoons of basil pesto into each pocket of the chicken breasts, spreading it evenly.

5. Place a slice of mozzarella cheese on top of the pesto in each chicken breast pocket.

6. Gently press the edges of the chicken breasts together to seal the pockets.

7. Heat olive oil in an oven-safe skillet over medium-high heat.

8. Sear the chicken breasts in the skillet for about 3-4 minutes per side until they develop a golden brown crust.

9. Transfer the skillet to the preheated oven and bake for 15-18 minutes or until the chicken is crough and no longer pink in the centre. The internal temperature should reach 165°F (74°C).

10. Remove the skillet from the oven and let the chicken breasts rest for a few minutes before serving.

11. Serve the pesto-stuffed chicken breasts hot with your favourite side dishes, such as roasted vegetables or a fresh salad.

Nutrition Facts: (Note: Nutritional values may vary depending on the specific ingredients and brands used.)

Serving Size: 1 stuffed chicken breast Calories: Approximately 300 Total Fat: 18g

• Saturated Fat: 6g

• Trans Fat: 0g Cholesterol: 90mg Sodium: 450mg Total Carbohydrate: 2g

• Dietary Fiber: 0g

• Sugars: 0g Protein: 33g

Please note that the nutrition facts are approximate and may vary based on the specific ingredients used and the serving size.

CINNAMON SUGAR APPLE CHIPS

Prep Time: 10 minutes Cooking Time: 2 hours Servings: 4

Ingredients:

• four large apples (any variety)
• two tablespoons granulated sugar
• one teaspoon ground cinnamon

Directions:

1. Preheat your oven to 225°F (110°C) and line two baking sheets with parchment paper.

2. Wash and core the apples. Using a sharp knife or a mandoline slicer, slice the apples into very thin rounds, about 1/8-inch thick. Try to make the slices as uniform as possible.

3. In a small bowl, combine the granulated sugar and ground cinnamon. Mix well.

4. Place the apple slices on the prepared baking sheets in a single, ensuring they do not overlap. Sprinkle the cinnamon sugar mixture evenly over the apple slices.

5. Place the baking sheets in the preheated oven and bake for about 2 hours or until the

apple slices are dry and crispy. The baking time may vary depending on the thickness of the slices, so keep an eye on them after the first hour.

6. Once the apple chips are crispy, remove them from the oven and allow them to cool completely on the baking sheets. They will become even crispier as they cool down.

7. Once cooled, transfer the cinnamon sugar apple chips to an airtight container or serve them immediately. They can be stored for up to a week, but they are best enjoyed fresh.

Nutrition Facts (per serving):
- Calories: 92
- Total Fat: 0.2g
- Saturated Fat: 0g
- Cholesterol: 0mg
- Sodium: 1mg
- Total Carbohydrate: 24g
- Dietary Fiber: 4g
- Sugars: 18g
- Protein: **0.4g**

Note: The nutrition facts are approximate and may vary depending on the specific ingredients used.

ASIAN SESAME CHICKEN WINGS

Prep Time: 10 minutes Cooking Time: 35 minutes Serving: 4

Ingredients:

- 2 pounds of chicken wings
- two tablespoons soy sauce
- two tablespoons hoisin sauce
- 2 tablespoons honey
- 2 tablespoons sesame oil
- two cloves garlic, minced
- one teaspoon grated ginger
- one tablespoon rice vinegar
- one tablespoon Sriracha sauce (optional)
- 2 tablespoons sesame seeds
- Salt and pepper to taste
- Chopped green onions for garnish

Directions:

1. Preheat your oven to 400°F (200°C) and line a baking sheet with parchment paper.

2. In a large bowl, combine soy sauce, hoisin sauce, honey, sesame oil, minced garlic, grated ginger, rice vinegar, Sriracha sauce (if using), sesame seeds, salt, and pepper. Mix well to make the marinade.

3. Add the chicken wings to the bowl with the marinade and toss to coat them evenly. Let them marinate for about 15 minutes.

4. Arrange the marinated chicken wings on the prepared baking sheet, making sure they are in a single layer.

5. Bake the wings in the preheated oven for 30-35 minutes or until they are cooked through and crispy. Flip the wings halfway through the cooking time for even browning.

6. Once cooked, remove the wings from the oven and transfer them to a serving platter. Garnish with chopped green onions.

7. Serve the Asian Sesame Chicken Wings hot as an appetizer or as part of a main course. They pair well with steamed rice and stir-fried vegetables.

Nutrition Facts (per serving): Calories: 340 Total Fat: 20g Saturated Fat: 5g Cholesterol: 95mg Sodium: 710mg Carbohydrates: 10g Fiber: 1g Sugar: 8g Protein: 29g

Note: Nutrition facts may vary depending on the specific ingredients and brands used.

CAPRESE STUFFED MUSHROOMS

Prep Time: 15 minutes Cooking Time: 20 minutes Servings: 4

Ingredients:

- 16 large white mushrooms
- 1 cup cherry tomatoes, halved

- 8 ounces fresh mozzarella cheese, diced
- ¼ cup fresh basil leaves, chopped
- Two cloves garlic, minced
- Two tablespoons of balsamic glaze
- Salt and pepper to taste
- Olive oil for drizzling

Directions:

1. Preheat your oven to 375°F (190°C). Line a baking sheet with parchment paper.

2. Remove the stems from the mushrooms and gently clean them with a damp cloth. Set them aside.

3. In a mixing bowl, combine the cherry tomatoes, mozzarella cheese, basil leaves, minced garlic, salt, and pepper. Mix well.

4. Take each mushroom cap and spoon the tomato and mozzarella mixture into it, filling it generously. Place the stuffed mushrooms on the prepared baking sheet.

5. Drizzle a little olive oil over each stuffed mushroom.

6. Bake in the preheated oven for about 20 minutes or until the mushrooms are tender and the cheese is melted and slightly golden.

7. Remove from the oven and drizzle the balsamic glaze over the stuffed mushrooms.

8. Serve the Caprese Stuffed Mushrooms as a delicious appetizer or side dish.

Nutrition Facts (per serving):

- Calories: 155
- Total Fat: 9g
- Saturated Fat: 5g
- Cholesterol: 29mg
- Sodium: 280mg
- Total Carbohydrate: 7g
- Dietary Fiber: 1g
- Sugars: 4g
- Protein: 11g

Enjoy your Caprese Stuffed Mushrooms!

COCONUT CURRY SHRIMP

Prep Time: 15 minutes Cooking Time: 20 minutes Serving: 4 servings

Ingredients:

- 1 lb (450g) shrimp, peeled and deveined

- One tablespoon of vegetable oil
- 1 onion, finely chopped
- Three cloves garlic, minced
- 1 tablespoon fresh ginger, grated
- Two tablespoons of curry powder
- 1 can (14 oz/400 ml) coconut milk
- 1 cup chicken or vegetable broth
- One tablespoon of fish sauce
- One tablespoon of brown sugar
- One red bell pepper, sliced
- 1 cup snow peas
- One lime, juiced
- Salt and pepper to taste
- Fresh cilantro for garnish
- Cooked rice for serving

Directions:

1. Heat the vegetable oil in a large skillet over medium heat. Add the chopped onion and sauté until softened, about 5 minutes. Stir in the minced garlic and grated ginger, and cook for another minute until fragrant.

2. Add the curry powder to the skillet and stir well to coat the onion mixture. Cook for a minute to release the flavours.

3. Pour in the coconut milk and chicken or vegetable broth, and stir in the fish sauce and brown sugar. Bring the mixture to a simmer.

4. Add the shrimp to the skillet and cook for about 3-4 minutes, until they turn pink and are cooked through. Be careful not to overcook them, as they can become tough.

5. Stir in the sliced red bell pepper and snow peas, and cook for 2-3 minutes, until the vegetables are crisp-tender.

6. Squeeze the lime juice over the curry and season with salt and pepper to taste. Stir everything together.

7. Remove the skillet from heat and garnish with fresh cilantro.

8. Serve the Coconut Curry Shrimp over cooked rice.

Nutrition Facts (per serving):

- Calories: 320
- Fat: 18g
- Saturated Fat: 12g

- Cholesterol: 180mg
- Sodium: 690mg
- Carbohydrates: 14g
- Fibre: 3g
- Sugar: 6g
- Protein: 26g

Enjoy your Coconut Curry Shrimp!

BAKED CRAB CAKES

Prep Time: 20 minutes Cooking Time: 25 minutes Serving: 4 servings

Ingredients:

- 1 pound lump crab meat
- 1/2 cup bread crumbs
- 1/4 cup mayonnaise
- 1/4 cup finely chopped red bell pepper
- 1/4 cup finely chopped green onions
- One large egg, lightly beaten
- Two tablespoons of Dijon mustard
- 1 tablespoon Worcestershire sauce
- One tablespoon of fresh lemon juice
- 1/4 teaspoon Old Bay seasoning

- Salt and pepper to taste
- Cooking spray

Directions:

1. Preheat the oven to 400°F (200°C). Line a baking sheet with parchment paper and set aside.

2. In a large mixing bowl, combine the lump crab meat, bread crumbs, mayonnaise, red bell pepper, green onions, egg, Dijon mustard, Worcestershire sauce, lemon juice, Old Bay seasoning, salt, and pepper. Gently mix everything until well combined.

3. Divide the mixture into eight equal portions and shape each portion into a patty.

4. Place the crab cakes onto the prepared baking sheet and lightly coat them with cooking spray. This will help them crisp up in the oven.

5. Bake the crab cakes in the preheated oven for about 20-25 minutes or until golden brown and cooked through.

6. Once baked, remove the crab cakes from the oven and let them cool for a few minutes before serving.

7. Serve the baked crab cakes with your favourite sauce or aioli. They can be enjoyed as an appetizer or as a main course.

Nutrition Facts (per serving):

- Calories: 250
- Fat: 12g
- Saturated Fat: 2g
- Cholesterol: 150mg
- Sodium: 600mg
- Carbohydrates: 9g
- Fibre: 1g
- Sugar: 2g
- Protein: 25g

Note: Nutrition facts may vary depending on the specific ingredients and brands used.

BUFFALO CAULIFLOWER PIZZA BITES

Prep Time: 15 minutes Cooking Time: 25 minutes Serving: 4 servings

Ingredients:

- One medium head of cauliflower

- 1 cup all-purpose flour
- 1 cup milk (or non-dairy milk for a vegan option)
- One teaspoon of garlic powder
- One teaspoon of onion powder
- 1/2 teaspoon salt
- 1/4 teaspoon black pepper
- 1/2 cup buffalo sauce
- 1/4 cup melted butter (or vegan butter)
- 1/2 cup shredded mozzarella cheese (or vegan cheese)
- Two green onions, chopped
- Ranch dressing or blue cheese dressing for dipping (optional)

Directions:

1. Preheat your oven to 450°F (230°C). Line a baking sheet with parchment paper or lightly grease it.

2. Cut the cauliflower into small florets. In a large bowl, whisk together the flour, milk, garlic powder, onion powder, salt, and black pepper until smooth. Add the cauliflower florets to the batter and toss to coat them evenly.

3. Arrange the cauliflower florets in a single layer on the prepared baking sheet. Bake for 20 minutes or until they become crispy and lightly golden.

4. In a separate bowl, combine the buffalo sauce and melted butter. Toss the baked cauliflower florets in the buffalo sauce mixture until they are evenly coated.

5. Return the cauliflower florets to the baking sheet and sprinkle the shredded mozzarella cheese on top. Bake for 5 minutes or until the cheese has melted and is bubbly.

6. Remove from the oven and sprinkle the chopped green onions over the pizza bites.

7. Serve the Buffalo Cauliflower Pizza Bites hot with a side of ranch or blue cheese dressing for dipping, if desired.

Nutrition Facts: Serving Size: 1/4 of the recipe Calories: 240 Total Fat: 9g Saturated Fat: 5g Cholesterol: 20mg Sodium: 1040mg Total Carbohydrate: 31g Dietary Fiber: 3g Total Sugars: 4g Protein: 9g

Note: The nutrition facts are approximate and may vary based on the specific ingredients used and serving size.

HERBED LEMON SALMON PATTIES

Prep Time: 15 minutes Cooking Time: 10 minutes Serving: 4 patties

Ingredients:

- One can (14.75 ounces) of pink or red salmon, drained and flaked
- 1/2 cup bread crumbs
- 1/4 cup finely chopped red onion
- Two tablespoons chopped fresh parsley
- One tablespoon of chopped fresh dill
- One teaspoon of lemon zest
- One tablespoon of lemon juice
- 1/2 teaspoon salt
- 1/4 teaspoon black pepper
- Two large eggs, beaten
- Two tablespoons of vegetable oil

Directions:

1. In a mixing bowl, combine the flaked salmon, bread crumbs, red onion, parsley, dill, lemon zest, lemon juice, salt, and black pepper. Mix well until all the ingredients are evenly incorporated.

2. Add the beaten eggs to the salmon mixture and stir until the mixture is moistened and holds together. Let it sit for a few minutes to allow the bread crumbs to absorb some moisture.

3. Shape the mixture into four equal-sized patties, about 1/2 inch thick. Place them on a plate or baking sheet lined with parchment paper.

4. Heat the vegetable oil in a large non-stick skillet over medium heat. Once the oil is hot, carefully place the salmon patties in the skillet. Cook for about 4-5 minutes on each side until golden brown and crispy.

5. Remove the patties from the skillet and place them on a paper towel-lined plate to absorb any excess oil.

6. Serve the Herbed Lemon Salmon Patties hot as a main dish or in burger buns as a delicious seafood burger. You can also serve them with a side salad or dipping sauce.

Nutrition Facts (per serving):

- Calories: 240
- Total Fat: 13g
- Saturated Fat: 2.5g

- Cholesterol: 125mg
- Sodium: 520mg
- Total Carbohydrate: 13g
- Dietary Fiber: 1g
- Sugars: 2g
- Protein: 18g

Note: The nutrition facts are approximate and may vary depending on the specific ingredients and brands used.

ZUCCHINI AND FETA FRITTERS

Prep Time: 15 minutes Cooking Time: 15 minutes Servings: 4

Ingredients:
- Two medium zucchini, grated
- One teaspoon salt
- 1/2 cup crumbled feta cheese
- 1/4 cup finely chopped fresh herbs (such as dill, parsley, or mint)
- Two cloves garlic, minced
- 1/4 cup all-purpose flour
- Two large eggs, beaten

- 1/4 teaspoon black pepper
- Two tablespoons olive oil for frying
- Greek yoghurt or sour cream for serving (optional)

Directions:

1. Place the grated zucchini in a colander and sprinkle with salt. Let it sit for about 10 minutes to release excess moisture. Then, squeeze out the liquid from the zucchini using your hands or a clean kitchen towel.

2. In a mixing bowl, combine the grated zucchini, feta cheese, chopped herbs, minced garlic, flour, beaten eggs, and black pepper. Mix well until all the ingredients are evenly incorporated.

3. Heat olive oil in a large skillet over medium heat.

4. Take about 2 tablespoons of the zucchini mixture and form it into a small patty. Place the patties in the hot skillet, flattening them slightly with a spatula. Cook for about 3-4 minutes on each side or until the cakes are golden brown and crispy.

5. Remove the cooked patties from the skillet and transfer them to a paper towel-lined plate to absorb any excess oil.

6. Repeat the process with the remaining zucchini mixture until all the fritters are cooked.

7. Serve the Zucchini and Feta Fritters warm as an appetizer or a side dish. You can also serve them with a dollop of Greek yoghurt or sour cream on top if desired.

Nutrition Facts (per serving): Calories: 180 Total Fat: 12g

- Saturated Fat: 4g
- Trans Fat: 0g Cholesterol: 95mg Sodium: 520mg Total Carbohydrate: 10g
- Dietary Fiber: 1g
- Sugars: 2g Protein: 9g Vitamin D: 10% Calcium: 15% Iron: 6% Potassium: 230mg

Note: Nutrition facts may vary depending on the specific ingredients and brands used.

SPINACH AND FETA STUFFED CHICKEN BREAST

Prep Time: 15 minutes Cooking Time: 25 minutes Servings: 4

Ingredients:

- Four boneless, skinless chicken breasts
- 1 cup frozen spinach, thawed and drained
- 1/2 cup crumbled feta cheese
- 1/4 cup sun-dried tomatoes, chopped
- Two cloves garlic, minced
- One tablespoon of olive oil
- One teaspoon of dried oregano
- Salt and pepper, to taste
- Toothpicks

Directions:

1. Preheat your oven to 400°F (200°C). Grease a baking dish and set it aside.

2. In a mixing bowl, combine the spinach, feta cheese, sun-dried tomatoes, minced garlic, olive oil, dried oregano, salt, and pepper. Mix well until all the ingredients are evenly incorporated.

3. Lay the chicken breasts flat on a cutting board. Use a sharp knife to cut a slit horizontally along the side of each

chicken breast, creating a pocket for stuffing.

4. Stuff each chicken breast with an equal amount of the spinach and feta mixture, pressing it gently to fill the pocket. Secure the opening with toothpicks to keep the filling intact.

5. Heat a skillet over medium-high heat. Add a drizzle of olive oil and sear the stuffed chicken breasts for about 2-3 minutes on each side until they turn golden brown.

6. Transfer the seared chicken breasts to the prepared baking dish and place it in the preheated oven. Bake for 18-20 minutes or until the chicken is cooked and no longer pink in the centre.

7. Once cooked, remove the chicken from the oven and let it rest for a few minutes. Remove the toothpicks before serving.

8. Serve the Spinach and Feta Stuffed Chicken Breast hot, accompanied by your choice of sides like roasted vegetables, rice, or a fresh salad.

Nutrition Facts (per serving):

- Calories: 280
- Fat: 11g

- Saturated Fat: 4g
- Cholesterol: 100mg
- Sodium: 420mg
- Carbohydrates: 4g
- Fibre: 1g
- Sugar: 2g
- Protein: 38g

Note: The nutrition facts are approximate and may vary based on the specific ingredients and quantities used.

SWEET AND SPICY KOREAN CHICKEN WINGS

Prep Time: 10 minutes Cooking Time: 40 minutes Serving: 4 servings

Ingredients:
- 2 pounds of chicken wings
- 1/4 cup soy sauce
- 1/4 cup gochujang (Korean chilli paste)
- Three tablespoons honey
- Two tablespoons of rice vinegar
- Two tablespoons of sesame oil

- Two cloves garlic, minced
- One teaspoon of grated ginger
- One tablespoon sesame seeds for garnish
- Two green onions, thinly sliced, for garnish

Directions:

1. Preheat the oven to 425°F (220°C). Line a baking sheet with parchment paper or foil.

2. In a large bowl, whisk together soy sauce, gochujang, honey, rice vinegar, sesame oil, garlic, and ginger to make the marinade.

3. Add the chicken wings to the bowl and toss until they are well coated with the marinade. Let them marinate for at least 30 minutes or overnight in the refrigerator.

4. Place the marinated chicken wings on the prepared baking sheet, leaving space between each wing. Reserve the remaining marinade.

5. Bake the chicken wings in the preheated oven for 20 minutes, then remove from the oven and flip them over. Brush the wings with the reserved marinade.

6. Return the wings to the oven and bake for 15-20 minutes or until they are cooked through and crispy.

7. Remove the chicken wings from the oven and transfer them to a serving platter. Sprinkle with sesame seeds and sliced green onions.

8. Serve the sweet and spicy Korean chicken wings hot as an appetizer or as a main dish with steamed rice and your favourite side dishes.

Nutrition Facts (per serving): Calories: 390 Total Fat: 24g Saturated Fat: 6g Cholesterol: 95mg Sodium: 890mg Total Carbohydrate: 16g Dietary Fiber: 1g Total Sugars: 11g Protein: 28g

Note: The nutrition facts provided are estimates and may vary based on the specific ingredients used and serving size.

MEDITERRANEAN STUFFED BELL PEPPERS

Prep Time: 20 minutes Cooking Time: 40 minutes Serving: 4

Ingredients:

- Four large bell peppers (any colour)
- 1 cup cooked quinoa
- 1 cup canned chickpeas, drained and rinsed
- 1 cup diced tomatoes
- 1/2 cup crumbled feta cheese
- 1/4 cup chopped Kalamata olives
- 1/4 cup chopped fresh parsley
- Two cloves garlic, minced
- Two tablespoons extra-virgin olive oil
- One teaspoon of dried oregano
- Salt and pepper to taste

Directions:

1. Preheat your oven to 375°F (190°C).
2. Slice off the tops of the bell peppers and remove the seeds and membranes. Set them aside.
3. In a large mixing bowl, combine the cooked quinoa, chickpeas, diced tomatoes, feta cheese, Kalamata olives, parsley, minced garlic, olive oil, dried oregano, salt, and pepper. Mix well to combine all the ingredients.
4. Stuff the bell peppers with the quinoa mixture, packing it tightly.

5. Place the stuffed bell peppers in a baking dish and cover it with foil.

6. Bake in the preheated oven for 30 minutes.

7. Remove the foil and continue baking for an additional 10 minutes or until the peppers are tender and the filling is heated through.

8. Once cooked, remove them from the oven and let them cool for a few minutes before serving.

9. Garnish with additional chopped parsley, if desired.

10. Serve the Mediterranean Stuffed Bell Peppers as a main course or a side dish. Enjoy!

Nutrition Facts (per serving):

- Calories: 290
- Fat: 13g
- Saturated Fat: 4g
- Cholesterol: 17mg
- Sodium: 553mg
- Carbohydrates: 34g
- Fibre: 9g
- Sugar: 8g

- Protein: 11g

Note: The nutrition facts are approximate and may vary based on the specific ingredients used.

GARLIC PARMESAN KNOTS

Prep Time: 15 minutes Cooking Time: 15 minutes Serving: 4 servings

Ingredients:

- One can of refrigerated pizza dough
- Four tablespoons unsalted butter melted
- Three cloves garlic, minced
- Two tablespoons fresh parsley, finely chopped
- 1/4 cup grated Parmesan cheese
- Salt, to taste
- Pepper, to taste

Directions:

1. Preheat the oven to 400°F (200°C). Line a baking sheet with parchment paper or lightly grease it.

2. Open the can of refrigerated pizza dough and unroll it onto a clean surface. Cut the dough into 8 equal strips.

3. Take each strip of dough and tie it into a knot. Place the knots on the prepared baking sheet, leaving some space between them.

4. In a small bowl, combine the melted butter, minced garlic, chopped parsley, grated Parmesan cheese, salt, and pepper. Stir well to combine.

5. Brush the garlic Parmesan mixture over the knots, coating each one evenly.

6. Place the baking sheet in the preheated oven and bake for 12-15 minutes or until the knots are golden brown and cooked through.

7. Once the knots are done, remove them from the oven and let them cool for a few minutes.

8. Serve the Garlic Parmesan Knots warm. They can be enjoyed as an appetizer, a side dish, or a delicious accompaniment to pasta dishes or soups.

Nutrition Facts (per serving):

- Calories: 250

- Total Fat: 13g
- Saturated Fat: 7g
- Cholesterol: 30mg
- Sodium: 520mg
- Total Carbohydrate: 25g
- Dietary Fiber: 1g
- Sugars: 2g
- Protein: 6g

Note: Nutrition facts are approximate and may vary depending on the ingredients used.

CRISPY FRIED PICKLES

Prep Time: 15 minutes Cooking Time: 10 minutes Servings: 4

Ingredients:
- One jar of dill pickle spears (about 16 spears)
- 1 cup all-purpose flour
- One teaspoon paprika
- 1/2 teaspoon garlic powder
- 1/2 teaspoon cayenne pepper (optional for added heat)

- 1/2 teaspoon salt
- 1/4 teaspoon black pepper
- 1 cup buttermilk
- Vegetable oil for frying
- Ranch dressing or your favourite dipping sauce for serving

Directions:

1. Drain the pickle spears from the jar and pat them dry with paper towels. Set aside.

2. In a shallow bowl, combine the flour, paprika, garlic powder, cayenne pepper (if using), salt, and black pepper. Mix well to combine.

3. Pour the buttermilk into another shallow bowl.

4. Heat vegetable oil in a deep frying pan or Dutch oven to about 375°F (190°C).

5. Take a pickle spear and dip it into the buttermilk, ensuring it's fully coated. Allow any excess buttermilk to drip off.

6. Roll the pickle spear in the flour mixture, ensuring it's evenly coated. Gently shake off any excess flour.

7. Place the coated pickle spear into the hot oil. Repeat the process with a few more

pickles, being careful not to overcrowd the pan.

8. Fry the pickles for about 2-3 minutes or until they turn golden brown and crispy. Flip them halfway through to ensure even cooking.

9. Once the pickles are crispy and golden, remove them from the oil using a slotted spoon or tongs and transfer them to a plate lined with paper towels to drain any excess oil.

10. Continue frying the remaining pickles in batches until they're all cooked.

11. Serve the crispy fried pickles hot with ranch dressing or your favourite dipping sauce.

Nutrition Facts (per serving):

- Calories: 210
- Fat: 10g
- Saturated Fat: 2g
- Cholesterol: 6mg
- Sodium: 780mg
- Carbohydrates: 25g
- Fibre: 2g
- Sugar: 3g

- Protein: 5g

Note: The nutrition facts provided are approximate and may vary depending on the specific ingredients and brands used.

COCONUT LIME SHRIMP SKEWERS

Prep Time: 20 minutes Cooking Time: 10 minutes Serving: 4

Ingredients:

- 1 pound (450g) large shrimp, peeled and deveined
- 1 cup shredded coconut
- One lime, zest and juice
- Two tablespoons fresh cilantro chopped
- Two tablespoons of olive oil
- One tablespoon of soy sauce
- One tablespoon honey
- 1/2 teaspoon salt
- 1/4 teaspoon black pepper
- Wooden skewers, soaked in water for 30 minutes

Directions:

1. Preheat your grill or grill pan over medium-high heat.

2. In a large bowl, combine the shredded coconut, lime zest, and chopped cilantro. Mix well.

3. In a separate bowl, whisk together the olive oil, lime juice, soy sauce, honey, salt, and black pepper to make the marinade.

4. Add the shrimp to the marinade and toss until they are well coated. Allow the shrimp to marinate for about 10 minutes.

5. Thread the marinated shrimp onto the soaked wooden skewers.

6. Place the shrimp skewers on the preheated grill or grill pan and cook for about 3-4 minutes per side or until they turn pink and opaque.

7. While grilling, brush the remaining marinade onto the shrimp skewers for extra flavour.

8. Once the shrimp are cooked through, remove them from the grill and let them rest for a few minutes.

9. Serve the Coconut Lime Shrimp Skewers with a squeeze of fresh lime juice and garnish with additional cilantro, if desired.

Nutrition Facts (per serving):

- Calories: 250
- Fat: 15g
- Carbohydrates: 9g
- Protein: 20g
- Fibre: 2g

Note: The nutrition facts are approximate and may vary depending on the ingredients used.

BACON-WRAPPED STUFFED DATES

Prep Time: 15 minutes Cooking Time: 20 minutes Serving: 4

Ingredients:

- 12 Medjool dates
- Six slices of bacon, cut in half
- 4 ounces (115g) of goat cheese
- 1/4 cup (60ml) of honey
- Freshly ground black pepper

Directions:

1. Preheat your oven to 375°F (190°C) and line a baking sheet with parchment paper.

2. Make a lengthwise slit in each date and remove the pit.

3. Take a small amount of goat cheese and stuff it into each date.

4. Wrap each stuffed date with a half slice of bacon and secure it with a toothpick.

5. Arrange the bacon-wrapped dates on the prepared baking sheet.

6. Drizzle the honey over the dates and sprinkle with freshly ground black pepper.

7. Place the baking sheet in the preheated oven and bake for about 20 minutes or until the bacon is crispy and the cheese is melted.

8. Remove from the oven and let them cool for a few minutes.

9. Serve the bacon-wrapped stuffed dates warm as an appetizer or a delicious snack.

Nutrition Facts (per serving):

- Calories: 210
- Fat: 8g
- Saturated Fat: 4g
- Cholesterol: 20mg
- Sodium: 170mg

- Carbohydrates: 33g
- Fibre: 3g
- Sugar: 29g
- Protein: 4g

Enjoy your tasty Bacon-Wrapped Stuffed Dates!

LEMON HERB TILAPIA FILLETS

Prep Time: 10 minutes Cooking Time: 15 minutes Serving: 4

Ingredients:

- Four tilapia fillets
- Two lemons
- Three tablespoons olive oil
- Two tablespoons fresh parsley, chopped
- One tablespoon fresh dill, chopped
- One teaspoon dried thyme
- Salt and pepper to taste

Directions:

1. Preheat your oven to 400°F (200°C).
2. Rinse the tilapia fillets under cold water and pat them dry with paper towels.

3. Place the tilapia fillets in a single layer in a baking dish or on a baking sheet lined with parchment paper.

4. Cut one lemon in half and squeeze the juice over the tilapia fillets, distributing it evenly.

5. Drizzle the olive oil over the fillets.

6. Sprinkle the chopped parsley, dill, dried thyme, salt, and pepper over the fillets. Make sure to season both sides.

7. Slice the remaining lemon into thin rounds and place them on top of the fillets.

8. Bake the tilapia fillets in the preheated oven for about 12-15 minutes or until the fish is opaque and flakes easily with a fork.

9. Once cooked, remove the fillets from the oven and let them rest for a few minutes.

10. Serve the Lemon Herb Tilapia Fillets warm with the roasted lemon slices on top. You can garnish with additional fresh herbs if desired.

Nutrition Facts (per serving):

- Calories: 180
- Total Fat: 10g

- Saturated Fat: 2g
- Cholesterol: 55mg
- Sodium: 70mg
- Carbohydrates: 4g
- Fibre: 1g
- Sugar: 1g
- Protein: 20g

Note: The nutrition facts are approximate and may vary depending on the ingredients used.

CRISPY BRUSSELS SPROUTS WITH BALSAMIC GLAZE

Prep Time: 10 minutes Cooking Time: 25 minutes Serving: 4

Ingredients:
- 1 pound Brussels sprouts
- Two tablespoons olive oil
- Salt and pepper, to taste
- 1/4 cup balsamic glaze
- Two tablespoons honey (optional for extra sweetness)

- 1/4 cup grated Parmesan cheese (optional for garnish)

Directions:

1. Preheat your oven to 400°F (200°C). Line a baking sheet with parchment paper or lightly grease it with oil.

2. Trim the ends of the Brussels sprouts and remove any outer leaves that are wilted or damaged. Cut larger sprouts in half, keeping smaller ones whole.

3. Place the Brussels sprouts in a large bowl and drizzle with olive oil. Toss them to coat evenly. Season with salt and pepper to taste.

4. Spread the Brussels sprouts in a single layer on the prepared baking sheet. Make sure they are not overcrowded to ensure even browning.

5. Roast the Brussels sprouts in the preheated oven for about 20-25 minutes, or until they are crispy and browned, flipping them once halfway through.

6. While the Brussels sprouts are roasting, in a small saucepan, heat the balsamic glaze over low heat until warmed. If desired, add honey for extra sweetness and stir until well combined.

7. Once the Brussels sprouts are done, remove them from the oven and transfer them to a serving dish.

8. Drizzle the warm balsamic glaze over the roasted Brussels sprouts.

9. If desired, sprinkle grated Parmesan cheese over the top as a garnish.

10. Serve the crispy Brussels sprouts immediately as a delicious side dish or appetizer.

Nutrition Facts: The nutrition information may vary based on the specific ingredients used and any additional toppings or modifications made to the recipe. Here's a general overview:

Serving Size: 1/4 of the recipe Calories: Approximately 150 Total Fat: 8g Saturated Fat: 2g Cholesterol: 5mg Sodium: 200mg Carbohydrates: 16g Fiber: 4g Sugar: 8g Protein: 5g

Please note that these values are approximate and can vary depending on the specific ingredients and brands used.

CAJUN POPCORN SHRIMP

Prep Time: 20 minutes Cooking Time: 10 minutes Serving: 4 servings

Ingredients:

- 1 pound (450g) medium-sized shrimp, peeled and deveined
- 1 cup all-purpose flour
- One tablespoon Cajun seasoning
- One teaspoon garlic powder
- One teaspoon paprika
- 1/2 teaspoon salt
- 1/4 teaspoon black pepper
- Two large eggs
- Vegetable oil for frying
- Lemon wedges for serving
- Fresh parsley, chopped (optional), for garnish

Directions:

1. In a shallow bowl, whisk together the flour, Cajun seasoning, garlic powder, paprika, salt, and black pepper. Set aside.
2. In another shallow bowl, beat the eggs until well combined.
3. Dip each shrimp into the beaten eggs, allowing any excess to drip off, and then

coat it evenly with the flour mixture. Place the coated shrimp on a plate or baking sheet.

4. In a large, deep skillet or pot, heat about 1 inch (2.5cm) of vegetable oil over medium-high heat until it reaches 350°F (175°C).

5. Carefully add the coated shrimp to the hot oil in batches, making sure not to overcrowd the pan. Fry the shrimp for about 2-3 minutes or until they turn golden brown and crispy. Flip them halfway through for even cooking. Remove the cooked shrimp using a slotted spoon and transfer them to a plate lined with paper towels to drain excess oil.

6. Repeat the frying process with the remaining shrimp.

7. Once all the shrimp are cooked and drained, transfer them to a serving platter. Squeeze fresh lemon juice over the shrimp and garnish with chopped parsley if desired.

8. Serve the Cajun Popcorn Shrimp immediately as an appetizer or main dish. They are delicious on their own, but

you can also serve them with your favourite dipping sauce.

Nutrition Facts (per serving):

- Calories: 310
- Fat: 10g
- Saturated Fat: 2g
- Cholesterol: 260mg
- Sodium: 640mg
- Carbohydrates: 25g
- Fibre: 1g
- Sugar: 1g
- Protein: 28g

Note: The nutrition facts provided are estimates and may vary based on the specific ingredients used.

STUFFED BELL PEPPER RINGS

Prep Time: 15 minutes Cooking Time: 25 minutes Serving: 4 servings

Ingredients:

- Four large bell peppers (any colour)
- One tablespoon olive oil

- One small onion, diced
- Two cloves garlic, minced
- 1 pound ground beef (or any ground meat of your choice)
- 1 cup cooked rice
- 1 cup tomato sauce
- One teaspoon dried oregano
- One teaspoon dried basil
- 1/2 teaspoon salt
- 1/4 teaspoon black pepper
- 1 cup shredded mozzarella cheese
- Fresh parsley, chopped (for garnish)

Directions:

1. Preheat your oven to 375°F (190°C).

2. Cut the tops off the bell peppers and remove the seeds and membranes. Slice each bell pepper into 1-inch rings.

3. Heat olive oil in a large skillet over medium heat. Add diced onions and minced garlic, and sauté until the onions are translucent.

4. Add the ground beef to the skillet and cook until browned, breaking it up with a spoon as it cooks. Drain any excess fat.

5. Stir in the cooked rice, tomato sauce, dried oregano, dried basil, salt, and black pepper. Cook for another 2-3 minutes until well combined.

6. Place the bell pepper rings in a baking dish and fill each with the beef and rice mixture. Press the mixture down gently to compact it.

7. Cover the baking dish with foil and bake in the oven for 20 minutes.

8. Remove the foil and sprinkle the shredded mozzarella cheese over the bell pepper rings. Return to the oven and bake for another 5 minutes or until the cheese is melted and bubbly.

9. Garnish with chopped fresh parsley before serving.

Nutrition Facts (per serving):

- Calories: 320
- Fat: 16g
- Carbohydrates: 19g
- Protein: 25g
- Fibre: 4g
- Sugar: 7g
- Sodium: 570mg

Note: The nutrition facts are approximate and may vary based on the specific ingredients used.

PESTO MOZZARELLA STUFFED TOMATOES

Prep Time: 15 minutes Cooking Time: 15 minutes Serving: 4 servings

Ingredients:

- Four large tomatoes
- 1 cup fresh basil leaves
- Two cloves garlic
- ¼ cup pine nuts
- ½ cup grated Parmesan cheese
- ¼ cup olive oil
- Salt and pepper to taste
- 8 ounces fresh mozzarella cheese, cut into small cubes
- Fresh basil leaves for garnish

Directions:

1. Preheat your oven to 375°F (190°C).
2. Slice off the tops of the tomatoes and gently scoop out the pulp and seeds using

a spoon. Be careful not to puncture or tear the tomato shells. Set the hollowed-out tomatoes aside.

3. In a food processor or blender, combine the fresh basil leaves, garlic, pine nuts, grated Parmesan cheese, olive oil, salt, and pepper. Process until smooth and well combined, creating a pesto sauce.

4. Take the hollowed-out tomatoes and spoon a generous amount of the pesto sauce into each one, filling them about three-fourths full.

5. Place the mozzarella cheese cubes on top of the pesto-filled tomatoes, gently pressing them down.

6. Arrange the stuffed tomatoes in a baking dish and bake in the preheated oven for about 15 minutes, or until the cheese is melted and bubbly and the tomatoes are slightly softened.

7. Remove from the oven and let the stuffed tomatoes cool for a few minutes. Garnish with fresh basil leaves.

8. Serve the Pesto Mozzarella Stuffed Tomatoes as an appetizer or side dish. They can be enjoyed warm or at room temperature.

Nutrition Facts (per serving):

- Calories: 235
- Total Fat: 20g
- Saturated Fat: 5g
- Cholesterol: 20mg
- Sodium: 260mg
- Total Carbohydrate: 7g
- Dietary Fiber: 2g
- Sugars: 3g
- Protein: 10g

Note: The nutrition facts are approximate and may vary depending on the specific ingredients and quantities used.

HONEY MUSTARD CHICKEN DRUMSTICKS

Prep Time: 10 minutes Cooking Time: 40 minutes Serving: 4 servings

Ingredients:

- Eight chicken drumsticks
- 1/4 cup Dijon mustard
- 1/4 cup honey
- Two tablespoons olive oil

- Two tablespoons soy sauce
- Two cloves garlic, minced
- One teaspoon paprika
- 1/2 teaspoon salt
- 1/4 teaspoon black pepper
- Fresh parsley, chopped (for garnish)

Directions:

1. Preheat your oven to 400°F (200°C) and line a baking sheet with foil or parchment paper.

2. In a bowl, whisk together the Dijon mustard, honey, olive oil, soy sauce, minced garlic, paprika, salt, and black pepper until well combined.

3. Place the chicken drumsticks in a large ziplock bag or a shallow dish. Pour the honey mustard marinade over the drumsticks, ensuring they are coated evenly. Let them marinate for at least 30 minutes or overnight in the refrigerator for maximum flavour.

4. Arrange the marinated drumsticks on the prepared baking sheet, spacing them out evenly. Pour any remaining marinade over the drumsticks.

5. Place the baking sheet in the preheated oven and bake for about 35-40 minutes, or until the chicken is cooked through and golden brown. You can also use a meat thermometer to ensure the internal temperature reaches 165°F (74°C).

6. Once the drumsticks are cooked, remove them from the oven and let them rest for a few minutes. Garnish with fresh chopped parsley.

7. Serve the Honey Mustard Chicken Drumsticks hot with your favourite sides, such as roasted potatoes, steamed vegetables, or a fresh salad.

Nutrition Facts (per serving): Prep Time: 15 minutes Cooking Time: 30 minutes Serving: 4

Ingredients:

- One medium cauliflower head
- Two eggs
- 2 cups shredded mozzarella cheese
- 1/4 cup grated Parmesan cheese
- One teaspoon dried oregano
- 1/2 teaspoon garlic powder
- 1/2 teaspoon salt
- 1/4 teaspoon black pepper

- Marinara sauce for serving

Directions:

1. Preheat your oven to 425°F (220°C). Line a baking sheet with parchment paper and set it aside.

2. Cut the cauliflower into florets and pulse them in a food processor until finely chopped, resembling rice.

3. Place the cauliflower in a microwave-safe bowl and microwave for 4-5 minutes until tender. Allow it to cool for a few minutes.

4. Once the cauliflower has cooled, transfer it to a clean kitchen towel or cheesecloth. Squeeze out as much moisture as possible. This step is important to ensure the breadsticks hold together.

5. In a mixing bowl, combine the cauliflower, eggs, 1 cup of shredded mozzarella cheese, Parmesan cheese, dried oregano, garlic powder, salt, and black pepper. Mix until well combined.

6. Transfer the mixture onto the prepared baking sheet. Use your hands to shape it into a rectangle or square, about 1/4 inch thick.

7. Bake in the preheated oven for 20-25 minutes or until the edges turn golden brown.

8. Remove the baking sheet from the oven and sprinkle the remaining 1 cup of shredded mozzarella cheese evenly over the top.

9. Return the baking sheet to the oven and bake for another 5 minutes or until the cheese is melted and bubbly.

10. Remove from the oven and let it cool for a few minutes. Cut the cauliflower breadsticks into strips or squares.

11. Serve the cheesy cauliflower breadsticks warm with marinara sauce for dipping.

Nutrition Facts (per serving):

- Calories: 200
- Total Fat: 12g
- Saturated Fat: 7g
- Cholesterol: 109mg
- Sodium: 555mg
- Total Carbohydrate: 8g
- Dietary Fiber: 3g

- Sugars: 3g
- Protein: 16g

Note: The nutrition facts are approximate and may vary depending on the specific ingredients and brands used.

- Calories: 345
- Fat: 17g
- Saturated Fat: 4g
- Cholesterol: 130mg
- Sodium: 778mg
- Carbohydrates: 17g
- Fibre: 0.5g
- Sugar: 15g
- Protein: 31g

Note: The nutrition facts are approximate and may vary depending on the specific ingredients and quantities used.

CHEESY CAULIFLOWER BREADSTICKS

Prep Time: 20 minutes Cooking Time: 30 minutes Serving: 4

Ingredients:

- One medium-sized cauliflower head
- Two eggs
- 2 cups shredded mozzarella cheese
- 1/2 cup grated Parmesan cheese
- Two teaspoons of dried oregano
- One teaspoon of garlic powder
- 1/2 teaspoon salt
- Marinara sauce for dipping (optional)

Directions:

1. Preheat your oven to 425°F (220°C). Line a baking sheet with parchment paper and set it aside.

2. Cut the cauliflower into florets, removing any large stems. Place the florets in a food processor and pulse until they resemble rice-like grains.

3. Transfer the cauliflower rice to a microwave-safe bowl and microwave on high for 5-6 minutes or until the

cauliflower is tender. Allow it to cool for a few minutes.

4. Once the cauliflower has cooled, place it in a clean kitchen towel or cheesecloth. Squeeze out any excess moisture over the sink until you have removed as much liquid as possible.

5. In a large mixing bowl, combine the cauliflower rice, eggs, shredded mozzarella cheese, grated Parmesan cheese, dried oregano, garlic powder, and salt. Mix everything well until a sticky dough forms.

6. Transfer the dough to the prepared baking sheet and spread it out evenly, shaping it into a rectangular or square shape.

7. Bake the cauliflower breadsticks in the preheated oven for about 25-30 minutes, or until they turn golden brown and the edges start to crisp up.

8. Once cooked, remove the breadsticks from the oven and allow them to cool for a few minutes. Then, using a sharp knife, slice them into breadstick-sized pieces.

9. Serve the Cheesy Cauliflower Breadsticks warm with a marinara sauce for dipping, if desired.

Nutrition Facts (per serving):

- Calories: 180
- Fat: 10g
- Saturated Fat: 6g
- Cholesterol: 101mg
- Sodium: 528mg
- Carbohydrates: 7g
- Fibre: 2g
- Sugar: 3g
- Protein: 16g

Note: Nutrition facts may vary depending on the specific brands of ingredients used and any modifications made to the recipe.

CILANTRO LIME CHICKEN SKEWERS

Prep Time: 15 minutes Cooking Time: 15 minutes Serving: 4 servings

Ingredients:

- 1.5 lbs (680g) boneless, skinless chicken breasts cut into 1-inch cubes

- 1/4 cup freshly squeezed lime juice
- 1/4 cup chopped fresh cilantro leaves
- Two tablespoons of olive oil
- Two cloves garlic, minced
- One teaspoon of ground cumin
- 1/2 teaspoon salt
- 1/4 teaspoon black pepper
- One red bell pepper, cut into chunks
- One green bell pepper, cut into chunks
- One red onion, cut into chunks

Directions:

1. In a large bowl, combine the lime juice, cilantro, olive oil, minced garlic, ground cumin, salt, and black pepper. Mix well to make the marinade.

2. Add the chicken cubes to the marinade and toss to coat them evenly. Allow the chicken to marinate for at least 30 minutes in the refrigerator or overnight for maximum flavour.

3. Preheat the grill or grill pan over medium-high heat.

4. Thread the marinated chicken, red bell pepper, green bell pepper, and red onion

onto skewers, alternating between the ingredients.

5. Place the skewers on the preheated grill and cook for about 6-8 minutes per side or until the chicken is cooked through and the vegetables are tender, rotating the skewers occasionally.

6. Remove the skewers from the grill and let them rest for a few minutes before serving.

7. Serve the cilantro lime chicken skewers hot with a side of rice, salad, or your favourite dipping sauce.

Nutrition Facts:

- Serving Size: 1 serving
- Calories: 280
- Total Fat: 10g
- Saturated Fat: 2g
- Cholesterol: 110mg
- Sodium: 350mg
- Carbohydrates: 9g
- Fibre: 2g
- Sugar: 4g
- Protein: 38g

Note: Nutrition facts may vary depending on the specific ingredients and quantities used.

COCONUT CURRY CHICKEN WINGS

Prep Time: 15 minutes Cooking Time: 40 minutes Serving: 4 servings

Ingredients:

- 2 pounds of chicken wings
- 1 cup coconut milk
- Two tablespoons of red curry paste
- Two tablespoons of fish sauce
- Two tablespoons of lime juice
- 2 tablespoons brown sugar
- One teaspoon of ground turmeric
- One teaspoon of ground cumin
- One teaspoon of ground coriander
- 1 teaspoon salt
- 1/2 teaspoon black pepper
- 2 tablespoons vegetable oil
- Fresh cilantro for garnish
- Lime wedges for serving

Directions:

1. Preheat the oven to 400°F (200°C). Line a baking sheet with parchment paper or foil.

2. In a large mixing bowl, combine coconut milk, red curry paste, fish sauce, lime juice, brown sugar, turmeric, cumin, coriander, salt, and black pepper. Mix well to create the marinade.

3. Add the chicken wings to the bowl and toss to coat them evenly with the marinade. Let them marinate for at least 30 minutes, or refrigerate overnight for maximum flavour.

4. Heat vegetable oil in a large skillet over medium-high heat. Remove the chicken wings from the marinade, shaking off any excess, and transfer them to the skillet. Cook the wings for about 5 minutes, turning occasionally, until they are browned on all sides.

5. Transfer the browned wings to the prepared baking sheet and place them in the oven. Bake for 30-35 minutes or until the chicken is cooked through and crispy.

6. Remove the wings from the oven and let them cool slightly. Garnish with fresh cilantro.

7. Serve the Coconut Curry Chicken Wings with lime wedges on the side for squeezing over the wings. Enjoy!

Nutrition Facts (per serving):

- Calories: 320
- Fat: 21g
- Saturated Fat: 11g
- Cholesterol: 78mg
- Sodium: 850mg
- Carbohydrates: 11g
- Fibre: 1g
- Sugar: 7g
- Protein: 22g

Please note that the nutrition facts are approximate and may vary depending on the specific ingredients and quantities used.

GREEK STYLE STUFFED MUSHROOMS

Prep Time: 20 minutes Cooking Time: 25 minutes Serving: 4 servings

Ingredients:

- 24 large mushrooms, stems removed and reserved

- One tablespoon olive oil
- One small onion, finely chopped
- Two cloves garlic, minced
- 1/2 cup chopped spinach
- 1/2 cup crumbled feta cheese
- 1/4 cup grated Parmesan cheese
- 1/4 cup bread crumbs
- Two tablespoons chopped fresh parsley
- Salt and pepper to taste

Directions:

1. Preheat the oven to 375°F (190°C).
2. Finely chop the mushroom stems and set aside.
3. Heat the olive oil in a skillet over medium heat. Add the chopped onion and garlic, and cook until softened and fragrant, about 5 minutes.
4. Add the chopped mushroom stems and spinach to the skillet. Cook for another 3-4 minutes or until the mushrooms release their moisture and the spinach wilts.
5. Remove the skillet from heat and let the mixture cool slightly.

6. In a bowl, combine the cooked mushroom mixture with the feta cheese, Parmesan cheese, bread crumbs, and chopped parsley. Season with salt and pepper to taste.

7. Stuff each mushroom cap with the filling mixture and place them on a baking sheet.

8. Bake in the preheated oven for 20-25 minutes or until the mushrooms are tender and the filling is golden brown.

9. Remove from the oven and let them cool for a few minutes before serving.

Nutrition Facts (per serving):

- Calories: 180
- Fat: 10g
- Saturated Fat: 4g
- Cholesterol: 20mg
- Sodium: 350mg
- Carbohydrates: 14g
- Fibre: 3g
- Sugar: 4g
- Protein: 10g
- Vitamin D: 0mcg
- Calcium: 150mg

- Iron: 1mg
- Potassium: 560mg

Enjoy your Greek Style Stuffed Mushrooms!

HERB-ROASTED TURKEY BREAST

Prep Time: 15 minutes Cooking Time: 1 hour 30 minutes Serving: 6-8 servings

Ingredients:
- One bone-in turkey breast (about 4-5 pounds)
- Four tablespoons unsalted butter, melted
- Three cloves garlic, minced
- Two tablespoons fresh thyme leaves, chopped
- Two tablespoons fresh rosemary leaves, chopped
- One tablespoon fresh sage leaves, chopped
- One teaspoon salt
- 1/2 teaspoon black pepper
- One lemon, sliced
- 1 cup chicken broth

Directions:

1. Preheat your oven to 350°F (175°C).

2. Mix the melted butter, minced garlic, thyme, rosemary, sage, salt, and black pepper in a small bowl.

3. Place the turkey breast on a rack in a roasting pan. Pat it dry with paper towels.

4. Rub the herb butter mixture all over the turkey breast, making sure to get it under the skin as well.

5. Place the lemon slices on top of the turkey breast.

6. Pour the chicken broth into the bottom of the roasting pan.

7. Cover the roasting pan with aluminium foil, making a tent-like shape for airflow.

8. Place the roasting pan in the preheated oven and roast for about 1 hour.

9. After 1 hour, remove the aluminium foil tent and continue roasting for an additional 30 minutes, or until the internal temperature of the turkey breast reaches 165°F (74°C) when measured with a meat thermometer.

10. Once the turkey breast is cooked, remove it from the oven and let it rest for about 10 minutes before slicing.

11. Serve the herb-roasted turkey breast slices with the pan juices and any desired side dishes.

Nutrition Facts (per serving):

- Calories: 280
- Fat: 11g
- Saturated Fat: 5g
- Cholesterol: 135mg
- Sodium: 580mg
- Carbohydrates: 2g
- Protein: 42g

Note: Nutrition facts are approximate and may vary based on the size of the turkey breast and the specific ingredients used.

Enjoy your delicious Herb-Roasted Turkey Breast!

PARMESAN RANCH ZUCCHINI FRIES

Prep Time: 15 minutes Cooking Time: 20 minutes Serving: 4 servings

Ingredients:

- Two medium zucchinis
- 1/2 cup grated Parmesan cheese
- 1/2 cup bread crumbs
- 1 tablespoon dried ranch seasoning
- 1/2 teaspoon garlic powder
- 1/4 teaspoon salt
- 1/4 teaspoon black pepper
- Two large eggs

Directions:

1. Preheat your oven to 425°F (220°C). Line a baking sheet with parchment paper or lightly grease it.

2. Cut the zucchini into long, thin strips resembling French fries. Make sure they are roughly the same size to ensure even cooking.

3. In a shallow bowl or plate, combine the grated Parmesan cheese, bread crumbs, dried ranch seasoning, garlic powder, salt, and black pepper. Mix well to evenly distribute the seasonings.

4. In a separate bowl, beat the eggs until well combined.

5. Dip each zucchini strip into the beaten eggs, allowing any excess to drip off. Then, roll the zucchini strip in the Parmesan breadcrumb mixture, ensuring it is evenly coated. Place the coated zucchini strip on the prepared baking sheet. Repeat with the remaining zucchini strips.

6. Bake the zucchini fries in the oven for about 18-20 minutes or until they are golden brown and crispy. Flip the fries halfway through the baking time to ensure even browning.

7. Once the zucchini fries are cooked, remove them from the oven and let them cool for a few minutes before serving.

8. Serve the Parmesan Ranch Zucchini Fries with your favourite dipping sauce, such as ranch dressing, marinara sauce, or garlic aioli.

Nutrition Facts (per serving):

- Calories: 145
- Fat: 6g
- Saturated Fat: 2g
- Cholesterol: 96mg
- Sodium: 500mg

- Carbohydrates: 13g
- Fibre: 2g
- Sugar: 3g
- Protein: 9g

Note: The nutrition facts are approximate and may vary depending on the specific ingredients and brands used.

BBQ BACON-WRAPPED SHRIMP

Prep Time: 20 minutes Cooking Time: 10 minutes Serving: 4

Ingredients:

- 1 pound large shrimp, peeled and deveined
- Eight slices bacon, cut in half
- 1/4 cup barbecue sauce
- Two tablespoons brown sugar
- One teaspoon smoked paprika
- 1/2 teaspoon garlic powder
- Salt and black pepper, to taste
- Wooden skewers soaked in water

Directions:

1. Preheat your grill to medium-high heat.

2. In a small bowl, combine the barbecue sauce, brown sugar, smoked paprika, garlic powder, salt, and black pepper. Stir well to make the basting sauce.

3. Take each shrimp and wrap it with a half-slice of bacon. Secure the bacon in place with a wooden skewer.

4. Brush the bacon-wrapped shrimp with the basting sauce, coating them evenly.

5. Place the shrimp skewers on the preheated grill and cook for about 5 minutes per side until the bacon is crispy and the shrimp is opaque and cooked through. Baste the shrimp with the sauce occasionally while cooking.

6. Once cooked, remove the shrimp skewers from the grill and let them rest for a few minutes.

7. Serve the BBQ bacon-wrapped shrimp as an appetizer or as part of a main dish. They pair well with a side of coleslaw or grilled vegetables.

Nutrition Facts (per serving): Calories: 250 Fat: 12g Saturated Fat: 4g Cholesterol: 150mg Sodium: 780mg Carbohydrates: 12g Fiber: 0g Sugar: 10g Protein: 23g

Note: The nutrition facts are approximate and may vary depending on the specific ingredients and quantities used.

BUFFALO CHICKEN MEATBALLS

Prep Time: 15 minutes Cooking Time: 25 minutes Serving: 4 servings

Ingredients:

- 1 pound ground chicken
- 1/2 cup breadcrumbs
- 1/4 cup finely chopped celery
- 1/4 cup finely chopped green onions
- 1/4 cup crumbled blue cheese
- 1/4 cup hot sauce (such as Frank's RedHot)
- One large egg, lightly beaten
- 1/2 teaspoon garlic powder
- 1/2 teaspoon onion powder
- Salt and pepper to taste
- Ranch or blue cheese dressing for serving (optional)
- Celery sticks for serving (optional)

Directions:

1. Preheat your oven to 375°F (190°C) and line a baking sheet with parchment paper.

2. In a large bowl, combine the ground chicken, breadcrumbs, celery, green onions, blue cheese, hot sauce, egg, garlic powder, onion powder, salt, and pepper. Mix well until all ingredients are evenly incorporated.

3. Shape the mixture into meatballs about 1 inch in diameter, and place them on the prepared baking sheet.

4. Bake the meatballs in the preheated oven for about 20-25 minutes or until golden brown.

5. Remove the meatballs from the oven and let them cool slightly.

6. Serve the Buffalo Chicken Meatballs with ranch or blue cheese dressing on the side, if desired, and garnish with celery sticks for an extra crunch.

7. Enjoy your delicious Buffalo Chicken Meatballs!

Nutrition Facts: Serving Size: 4 meatballs Calories: 245 Total Fat: 12g

- Saturated Fat: 4g
- Trans Fat: 0g Cholesterol: 130mg Sodium: 560mg Total Carbohydrate: 10g
- Dietary Fiber: 1g
- Sugars: 1g Protein: 23g

Please note that the nutrition facts may vary based on the specific brands of ingredients used and any optional toppings or dressings.

ITALIAN STUFFED ZUCCHINI BOATS

Prep Time: 20 minutes Cooking Time: 30 minutes Servings: 4

Ingredients:
- Two large zucchinis
- One tablespoon olive oil
- One small onion, finely chopped
- Two cloves garlic, minced
- 1/2 pound ground beef or turkey
- 1 cup marinara sauce
- 1/2 teaspoon dried oregano
- 1/2 teaspoon dried basil
- Salt and pepper to taste

- 1 cup shredded mozzarella cheese
- Fresh basil leaves for garnish

Directions:

1. Preheat your oven to 375°F (190°C).
2. Cut the zucchinis in half lengthwise and scoop out the centres, creating a hollow "boat" shape. Chop the scooped-out zucchini flesh and set aside.
3. Heat olive oil in a large skillet over medium heat. Add the chopped onion, minced garlic, and sauté until they become soft and translucent.
4. Add the ground beef or turkey to the skillet, breaking it up with a spoon, and cook until browned and cooked through. Drain any excess fat if necessary.
5. Stir in the chopped zucchini flesh, marinara sauce, dried oregano, basil, salt, and pepper. Simmer the mixture for about 5 minutes to allow the flavours to meld together.
6. Place the hollowed-out zucchini boats in a baking dish, and spoon the meat mixture evenly into each boat.
7. Cover the baking dish with foil and bake in the oven for 20 minutes.

8. Remove the foil and sprinkle shredded mozzarella cheese over the top of each boat. Return the dish to the oven and bake uncovered for 10 minutes or until the cheese is melted and bubbly.

9. Once cooked, remove the zucchini boats from the oven and let them cool slightly. Garnish with fresh basil leaves.

10.   Serve the Italian Stuffed Zucchini Boats hot, and enjoy!

Nutrition Facts (per serving):

- Calories: 280
- Fat: 15g
- Carbohydrates: 11g
- Fibre: 3g
- Protein: 24g

Note: The nutrition facts may vary depending on the specific ingredients and brands used.

SPICY SRIRACHA TOFU BITES

Prep Time: 15 minutes Cooking Time: 20 minutes Serving: 4

Ingredients:

- One block of firm tofu
- Three tablespoons soy sauce
- Two tablespoons sriracha sauce
- Two tablespoons maple syrup
- One tablespoon rice vinegar
- 2 cloves garlic, minced
- One teaspoon grated ginger
- 1/4 cup cornstarch
- 2 tablespoons vegetable oil
- Sesame seeds, for garnish
- Chopped green onions for garnish

Directions:

1. Start by pressing the tofu to remove excess moisture. Place the tofu block on a plate lined with paper towels. Put another layer of paper towels on top and place a heavy object, such as a book or a pan, on top of the tofu. Let it sit for about 10 minutes.

2. While the tofu is being pressed, prepare the sauce. In a small bowl, whisk together soy sauce, sriracha sauce, maple syrup, rice vinegar, minced garlic, and grated ginger. Set aside.

3. After pressing the tofu, cut it into bite-sized cubes.

4. In a shallow dish, spread out the cornstarch. Roll the tofu cubes in the cornstarch until they are evenly coated.

5. Heat the vegetable oil in a large skillet over medium heat. Add the tofu cubes and cook for about 5 minutes, flipping them occasionally, until they become golden and crispy.

6. Once the tofu is cooked, pour the sauce over the tofu in the skillet. Stir gently to coat the tofu evenly with the sauce. Cook for 2-3 minutes, allowing the sauce to thicken and coat the tofu.

7. Remove the skillet from heat and let the tofu bites cool slightly. Sprinkle with sesame seeds and chopped green onions for garnish.

8. Serve the Spicy Sriracha Tofu Bites as an appetizer or a main course with steamed rice or noodles.

Nutrition Facts (per serving):

- Calories: 220
- Total Fat: 11g
- Saturated Fat: 1.5g

- Cholesterol: 0mg
- Sodium: 980mg
- Total Carbohydrate: 20g
- Dietary Fiber: 1g
- Sugars: 8g
- Protein: 12g

Please note that the nutrition facts are approximate and may vary depending on the specific ingredients and quantities used.

CAPRESE CHICKEN SKEWERS

Prep Time: 15 minutes Cooking Time: 15 minutes Serving: 4 servings

Ingredients:
- 1 pound boneless, skinless chicken breasts
- Two tablespoons olive oil
- Two teaspoons Italian seasoning
- Salt and pepper to taste
- Eight small mozzarella balls (or fresh mozzarella, cut into small cubes)
- Eight cherry tomatoes

- Fresh basil leaves
- Balsamic glaze (optional for serving)

Directions:

1. Preheat your grill or grill pan to medium-high heat.

2. Cut the chicken breasts into bite-sized pieces, about 1 inch in size.

3. In a bowl, combine the olive oil, Italian seasoning, salt, and pepper. Mix well.

4. Add the chicken pieces to the bowl and toss until they are evenly coated with the seasoning mixture.

5. Thread the chicken, mozzarella balls, cherry tomatoes, and basil leaves onto skewers, alternating the ingredients.

6. Place the skewers on the preheated grill and cook for about 5-7 minutes per side, or until the chicken is cooked through and the cheese is slightly melted.

7. Remove the skewers from the grill and let them rest for a few minutes.

8. Serve the Caprese chicken skewers on a platter, drizzle with balsamic glaze if desired, and garnish with additional fresh basil leaves.

Nutrition Facts (per serving):

- Calories: 280
- Fat: 15g
- Saturated Fat: 6g
- Cholesterol: 85mg
- Sodium: 300mg
- Carbohydrates: 2g
- Fibre: 0g
- Sugar: 1g
- Protein: 33g

Note: The nutrition facts are approximate and may vary depending on the specific ingredients used. The balsamic glaze is optional and can add additional calories and carbohydrates.

SPINACH AND FETA STUFFED MUSHROOMS

Prep Time: 15 minutes Cooking Time: 25 minutes Serving: 4

Ingredients:

- 16 large mushrooms
- 2 cups fresh spinach, chopped
- 1/2 cup crumbled feta cheese

- 1/4 cup grated Parmesan cheese
- Two cloves garlic, minced
- Two tablespoons olive oil
- One tablespoon fresh lemon juice
- Salt and pepper to taste

Directions:

1. Preheat the oven to 375°F (190°C). Lightly grease a baking dish.

2. Remove the stems from the mushrooms and set them aside. Place the mushroom caps in the greased baking dish and gill side up.

3. Finely chop the mushroom stems and set them aside.

4. In a skillet, heat the olive oil over medium heat. Add the chopped mushroom stems and minced garlic, and sauté for 3-4 minutes until the mushrooms are tender.

5. Add the chopped spinach to the skillet and cook for another 2-3 minutes, until the spinach has wilted. Remove from heat.

6. In a bowl, combine the cooked mushroom stems and spinach mixture with the crumbled feta cheese, grated

Parmesan cheese, and lemon juice. Stir well to combine.

7. Season the mixture with salt and pepper to taste.

8. Spoon the filling into each mushroom cap, pressing it down gently.

9. Bake the stuffed mushrooms in the preheated oven for 20-25 minutes, until the mushrooms are tender and the filling is golden brown.

10.   Remove from the oven and let them cool for a few minutes before serving.

11.   Serve the Spinach and Feta Stuffed Mushrooms as an appetizer or side dish.

Nutrition Facts (per serving):

- Calories: 142
- Fat: 10g
- Saturated Fat: 4g
- Cholesterol: 17mg
- Sodium: 273mg
- Carbohydrates: 7g
- Fibre: 2g
- Sugar: 2g
- Protein: 7g

Note: Nutrition facts may vary depending on the specific ingredients used.

LEMON GARLIC HERB TILAPIA

Prep Time: 10 minutes Cooking Time: 15 minutes Servings: 4

Ingredients:

- Four tilapia fillets
- Two tablespoons olive oil
- Two cloves garlic, minced
- One lemon, zested and juiced
- 1 teaspoon dried oregano
- One teaspoon dried thyme
- Salt and pepper to taste
- Fresh parsley, chopped (for garnish)

Directions:

1. Preheat the oven to 400°F (200°C). Grease a baking dish with a little olive oil, or use parchment paper to line it.
2. Place the tilapia fillets in the prepared baking dish, ensuring they are not overlapping.

3. In a small bowl, combine the olive oil, minced garlic, lemon zest, lemon juice, dried oregano, dried thyme, salt, and pepper. Mix well to create a marinade.

4. Pour the marinade over the tilapia fillets, ensuring they are evenly coated. Let them marinate for about 5 minutes to absorb the flavours.

5. Bake the tilapia in the preheated oven for 12-15 minutes or until the fish is cooked and flakes easily with a fork.

6. Once cooked, remove the tilapia from the oven and garnish with fresh parsley.

7. Serve the Lemon Garlic Herb Tilapia hot with steamed vegetables, rice, or a salad for a complete meal.

Nutrition Facts (per serving):

- Calories: 180
- Fat: 8g
- Saturated Fat: 1g
- Cholesterol: 55mg
- Sodium: 70mg
- Carbohydrates: 2g
- Fibre: 1g
- Sugar: 0g

- Protein: 25g

Note: The nutrition facts are approximate and may vary based on the specific ingredients used.

CRISPY EGGPLANT FRIES

Prep Time: 20 minutes Cooking Time: 25 minutes Serving: 4 servings

Ingredients:

- One large eggplant
- 1 cup bread crumbs
- 1/2 cup grated Parmesan cheese
- Two teaspoons dried Italian seasoning
- One teaspoon garlic powder
- 1/2 teaspoon salt
- 1/4 teaspoon black pepper
- Two large eggs, beaten
- Cooking spray
- Marinara sauce or your preferred dipping sauce for serving

Directions:

1. Preheat the oven to 425°F (220°C). Line a baking sheet with parchment paper or aluminium foil and lightly coat it with cooking spray.

2. Cut the eggplant into long, thin strips resembling French fries. You can peel the eggplant if desired, but leaving the skin on adds texture.

3. In a shallow dish, combine the bread crumbs, grated Parmesan cheese, dried Italian seasoning, garlic powder, salt, and black pepper. Mix well.

4. Dip each eggplant strip into the beaten eggs, making sure to coat it completely. Then, roll the egg-coated strip in the breadcrumb mixture, pressing gently to help the crumbs adhere. Place the coated strip on the prepared baking sheet. Repeat with the remaining eggplant strips.

5. Lightly coat the coated eggplant strips with cooking spray. This will help them crisp up in the oven.

6. Bake the eggplant fries in the preheated oven for about 20-25 minutes or until they are golden brown and crispy. Flip

them over halfway through the cooking time to ensure even browning.

7. Once the eggplant fries are done, remove them from the oven and let them cool for a few minutes. Serve them hot with marinara sauce or your preferred dipping sauce.

Nutrition Facts (per serving):

- Calories: 180
- Fat: 7g
- Saturated Fat: 3g
- Cholesterol: 100mg
- Sodium: 550mg
- Carbohydrates: 21g
- Fibre: 5g
- Sugar: 6g
- Protein: 10g

Note: The nutrition facts are approximate and may vary based on the specific ingredients and brands used.

CAJUN GARLIC BUTTER SHRIMP

Prep Time: 10 minutes Cooking Time: 10 minutes Servings: 4

Ingredients:

- 1 pound (450g) large shrimp, peeled and deveined
- 3 tablespoons unsalted butter
- Four cloves garlic, minced
- One teaspoon Cajun seasoning
- 1/2 teaspoon paprika
- 1/4 teaspoon cayenne pepper (optional for added heat)
- Salt and black pepper, to taste
- Two tablespoons fresh parsley, chopped
- Lemon wedges for serving

Directions:

1. In a large skillet, melt the butter over medium heat. Add the minced garlic and sauté for 1-2 minutes until fragrant.

2. Add the Cajun seasoning, paprika, and cayenne pepper (if using) to the skillet. Stir well to combine the spices with the butter and garlic.

3. Add the shrimp to the skillet and season with salt and black pepper to taste. Cook for 3-4 minutes, flipping the shrimp

halfway through until they turn pink and opaque.

4. Sprinkle the chopped parsley over the cooked shrimp and toss to coat them evenly with the garlic butter sauce.

5. Remove the skillet from heat. Serve the Cajun garlic butter shrimp hot with lemon wedges on the side for squeezing over the shrimp.

Nutrition Facts (per serving):

- Calories: 215
- Fat: 12g
- Saturated Fat: 6g
- Cholesterol: 260mg
- Sodium: 512mg
- Carbohydrates: 2g
- Fibre: 0.5g
- Sugar: 0.5g
- Protein: 24g

Note: The nutrition facts are approximate and may vary depending on the specific ingredients used.

BACON-WRAPPED SWEET POTATO WEDGES

Prep Time: 15 minutes Cooking Time: 30 minutes Serving: 4 servings

Ingredients:

- Two medium-sized sweet potatoes
- Eight slices of bacon
- Two tablespoons olive oil
- One teaspoon paprika
- 1/2 teaspoon garlic powder
- 1/2 teaspoon salt
- 1/4 teaspoon black pepper
- Fresh parsley, chopped (for garnish)

Directions:

1. Preheat your oven to 400°F (200°C) and line a baking sheet with parchment paper.

2. Wash and peel the sweet potatoes. Cut them into wedges, about 1/2-inch thick.

3. Mix the olive oil, paprika, garlic powder, salt, and black pepper in a small bowl.

4. Wrap each sweet potato wedge with a slice of bacon, securing it with a

toothpick if necessary. Place the wrapped wedges on the prepared baking sheet.

5. Brush the olive oil mixture over the bacon-wrapped sweet potato wedges, ensuring they are evenly coated.

6. Bake in the preheated oven for about 25-30 minutes or until the bacon is crispy and the sweet potatoes are tender.

7. Once cooked, remove the toothpicks if used and transfer the wedges to a serving plate.

8. Garnish with freshly chopped parsley for added freshness and colour.

9. Serve the bacon-wrapped sweet potato wedges hot as an appetizer or side dish.

Nutrition Facts (per serving):

- Calories: 235
- Total Fat: 16g
- Saturated Fat: 5g
- Cholesterol: 25mg
- Sodium: 630mg
- Total Carbohydrate: 17g
- Dietary Fiber: 2g
- Sugars: 5g
- Protein: 6g

Note: The nutrition facts are approximate and may vary depending on the ingredients used and portion sizes.

MEDITERRANEAN STUFFED CHICKEN BREAST

Prep Time: 15 minutes Cooking Time: 35 minutes Serving: 4 servings

Ingredients:

- Four boneless, skinless chicken breasts
- 1 cup cherry tomatoes, halved
- 1/2 cup chopped Kalamata olives
- 1/2 cup crumbled feta cheese
- 1/4 cup chopped fresh basil leaves
- Two tablespoons chopped fresh oregano leaves
- Two tablespoons extra-virgin olive oil
- Two cloves garlic, minced
- Salt and pepper, to taste

Directions:

1. Preheat the oven to 375°F (190°C).

2. Slice a pocket into each chicken breast by making a horizontal cut in the side, being careful not to cut all the way through.

3. In a bowl, combine the cherry tomatoes, Kalamata olives, feta cheese, basil, oregano, olive oil, garlic, salt, and pepper. Mix well to combine.

4. Spoon the tomato and olive mixture into the pockets of each chicken breast, dividing it evenly among them.

5. Use toothpicks to secure the openings of the chicken breasts.

6. Heat a large oven-safe skillet over medium-high heat. Add a drizzle of olive oil to the skillet.

7. Place the stuffed chicken breasts in the skillet and cook for 3-4 minutes on each side, until browned.

8. Transfer the skillet to the preheated oven and bake for 20-25 minutes, or until the chicken is cooked through and no longer pink in the centre.

9. Remove the toothpicks from the chicken breasts and let them rest for a few minutes before serving.

10.   Serve the Mediterranean stuffed chicken breasts with your favourite sides or a fresh salad.

Nutrition Facts (per serving):

- Calories: 320
- Fat: 14g
- Saturated Fat: 5g
- Cholesterol: 105mg
- Sodium: 550mg
- Carbohydrates: 7g
- Fibre: 2g
- Sugar: 3g
- Protein: 40g

Note: Nutrition facts may vary depending on the specific ingredients and brands used.

CHEESY SPINACH ARTICHOKE DIP

Prep Time: 15 minutes Cooking Time: 25 minutes Serving: 6-8 servings

Ingredients:

- 1 cup frozen spinach, thawed and drained

- 1 cup canned artichoke hearts, drained and chopped
- 1 cup shredded mozzarella cheese
- 1 cup grated Parmesan cheese
- 1 cup sour cream
- 1/2 cup mayonnaise
- 1/2 cup cream cheese, softened
- Three cloves garlic, minced
- 1/2 teaspoon dried oregano
- 1/2 teaspoon dried basil
- 1/2 teaspoon salt
- 1/4 teaspoon black pepper

Directions:

1. Preheat your oven to 350°F (175°C).

2. In a large mixing bowl, combine the thawed and drained spinach, chopped artichoke hearts, mozzarella cheese, Parmesan cheese, sour cream, mayonnaise, cream cheese, minced garlic, dried oregano, dried basil, salt, and black pepper. Mix well until all the ingredients are evenly combined.

3. Transfer the mixture to an oven-safe baking dish and spread it out evenly.

4. Place the baking dish in the preheated oven and bake for about 25 minutes or until the top is golden and bubbly.

5. Once done, remove the dip from the oven and let it cool for a few minutes before serving.

6. Serve the cheesy spinach artichoke dip warm with tortilla chips, bread slices, or vegetable sticks.

Nutrition Facts: (Serving Size: 1/8th of the recipe) Calories: 234 Total Fat: 19g

- Saturated Fat: 8g
- Trans Fat: 0g Cholesterol: 38mg Sodium: 565mg Total Carbohydrate: 7g
- Dietary Fiber: 2g
- Sugars: 2g Protein: 10g

Note: The nutrition facts are approximate and may vary based on the specific ingredients used.

TERIYAKI BEEF SKEWERS

Prep Time: 20 minutes Cooking Time: 10 minutes Serving: 4 servings

Ingredients:

- 1.5 pounds (680g) beef sirloin, cut into 1-inch cubes
- 1/2 cup soy sauce
- 1/4 cup mirin (sweet rice wine)
- 2 tablespoons brown sugar
- Two tablespoons rice vinegar
- Two cloves garlic, minced
- One teaspoon grated ginger
- One tablespoon cornstarch
- Two tablespoons water
- Bamboo skewers, soaked in water for 30 minutes

Directions:

1. In a bowl, combine soy sauce, mirin, brown sugar, rice vinegar, minced garlic, and grated ginger. Mix well to dissolve the sugar.

2. Place the beef cubes in a shallow dish or ziplock bag and pour the teriyaki marinade over them. Make sure all the beef pieces are coated. Marinate in the refrigerator for at least 1 hour or overnight for maximum flavour.

3. Preheat your grill or broiler.

4. In a small bowl, mix cornstarch and water to make a slurry. Set aside.

5. Thread the marinated beef cubes onto the soaked bamboo skewers.

6. Place the beef skewers on the grill or under the broiler and cook for 4-5 minutes on each side or until cooked to your desired doneness.

7. While the skewers are cooking, pour the remaining marinade into a small saucepan and boil over medium heat.

8. Once the marinade is boiling, reduce the heat and stir in the cornstarch slurry. Cook for an additional 1-2 minutes until the sauce thickens.

9. Remove the skewers from the grill or broiler and brush them with the thickened teriyaki sauce.

10. Serve the teriyaki beef skewers hot with steamed rice or a side of vegetables.

Nutrition Facts (per serving):

- Calories: 320
- Fat: 12g
- Carbohydrates: 12g
- Protein: 40g
- Sugar: 7g

- Sodium: 1030mg

Note: Nutrition facts may vary depending on the specific ingredients and brands used.

PESTO ZUCCHINI NOODLES

Prep Time: 15 minutes Cooking Time: 5 minutes Serving: 2 servings

Ingredients:

- Two large zucchini
- 1 cup fresh basil leaves
- 1/4 cup pine nuts
- Two cloves garlic, minced
- 1/4 cup grated Parmesan cheese
- 1/4 cup extra-virgin olive oil
- Salt and pepper to taste
- Cherry tomatoes (optional, for garnish)

Directions:

1. Use a spiralizer or julienne peeler to create long, thin zucchini noodles. Set aside.

2. In a food processor or blender, combine the fresh basil, pine nuts, minced garlic, and grated Parmesan cheese. Pulse a few

times until the ingredients are roughly chopped.

3. With the food processor running, slowly pour in the olive oil in a steady stream. Continue processing until the mixture forms a smooth pesto sauce. Add salt and pepper to taste.

4. Heat a large non-stick skillet over medium heat. Add the zucchini noodles to the skillet and cook for about 2-3 minutes, tossing them gently with tongs until tender.

5. Remove the skillet from heat and add the prepared pesto sauce to the zucchini noodles. Toss the noodles until they are well coated with the sauce.

6. Divide the Pesto Zucchini Noodles into two serving bowls. Garnish with cherry tomatoes, if desired.

7. Serve immediately and enjoy!

Nutrition Facts (per serving):

- Calories: 275
- Fat: 24g
- Carbohydrates: 8g
- Fibre: 3g
- Protein: 7g

Note: The nutrition facts are approximate and may vary depending on the specific ingredients used.

CONCLUSION

In conclusion, "Keto Air Fryer Cookbook for Beginners: Discover Delicious Low-Carb Recipes and Master the Art of Air Frying for Quick and Healthy Ketogenic Meals" is your ultimate companion for exploring the world of air frying. We've provided you with a diverse selection of recipes that will satisfy your cravings and keep you excited about cooking with your air fryer.

With this cookbook, you've discovered the incredible versatility of the air fryer and how it can transform your favourite dishes into healthier versions without sacrificing taste or texture. You've learned how to achieve that perfect golden crispness while retaining the juiciness and tenderness of your meals.

Whether you're a beginner or an experienced air fryer user, we've provided you with valuable tips, techniques, and cooking times to help you become a pro in the kitchen. You can now confidently experiment with various appetizers, main courses, sides, snacks, and even desserts, all made with the magic of air frying.

By incorporating these air fryer recipes into your daily cooking routine, you're treating yourself and your loved ones to delicious meals and making healthier choices. With reduced oil and a focus on fresh ingredients, you're embracing a lifestyle that promotes wellness and balance.

So, don't hesitate to embark on this exciting culinary journey. Open up "Keto Air Fryer Cookbook for Beginners" and let your creativity soar. From crispy and flavorful wings to innovative twists on classic favourites, you have a world of possibilities at your fingertips.

Thank you for joining us on this flavorful adventure. We hope this cookbook inspires you to continue exploring the endless possibilities of air frying and enjoying the delightful flavours of healthier meals. Happy air frying and bon appétit!

Made in United States
Orlando, FL
29 October 2024

53263914R00088